PIONEERING
BIONIC EAR
SURGEON

BILL GIBSON

WITHDRAWN FROM

G000146812

TINA K ALLEN BAppSc (Biomed), MA (Journalism), Dip Book
Publishing & Editing, worked as a medical scientist for ten years
before becoming a freelance medical writer and editor in 1996. She
has written feature stories for the GP magazine *Australian Doctor*,
edited the medical journal *Pathology* and most recently worked as the
consultant medical writer for Northside Clinic, part of Ramsay
Health Care. She was president of the Australasian Medical Writers
Association from 2005 to 2009. This is her first book. Tina lives with
her family on a farm in the Southern Highlands of New South Wales.

*This book is dedicated to my
husband David, my father Harold,
and my children James and Kaarina.*

PIONEERING
BIONIC EAR
SURGEON

BILL GIBSON

TINA K ALLEN

NEWSOUTH

A NewSouth book

Published by
NewSouth Publishing
University of New South Wales Press Ltd
University of New South Wales
Sydney NSW 2052
AUSTRALIA
newsouthpublishing.com

© Tina K Allen 2017
First published 2017

10 9 8 7 6 5 4 3 2 1

This book is copyright. Apart from any fair dealing for the purpose of private study, research, criticism or review, as permitted under the *Copyright Act*, no part of this book may be reproduced by any process without written permission. Inquiries should be addressed to the publisher.

National Library of Australia
Cataloguing-in-Publication entry
Creator: Allen, Tina K – author.
Title: Bill Gibson: Pioneering bionic ear surgeon / Tina K Allen.
ISBN: 9781742235301 (paperback)
    9781742248073 (ePDF)
    9781742242767 (ebook)
Notes: Includes bibliographical references and index.
Subjects: Gibson, Bill (William Peter Rea), 1944–
    Otolaryngologists—Australia—Biography.
    Surgeons—Australia—Biography.
    Otolaryngology—Australia.
    Cochlear implants—Australia.
    Ménière's disease—Australia.

Design Susanne Geppert
Cover design Luke Causby, Blue Cork
Cover photo Dr Gillian Dunlop
Printer Griffin Press

The information contained in this book is intended as general interest only. No information found here must under any circumstances be used for medical purposes, diagnostically, therapeutically or otherwise. If you, or anybody close to you, is affected, or believes he/she is affected, by any condition mentioned here, see a doctor. The author and publisher do not accept liability for anyone relying on the information in this book.

All reasonable efforts were taken to obtain permission to use copyright material reproduced in this book, but in some cases copyright could not be traced. The author welcomes information in this regard.

This book is printed on paper using fibre supplied from plantation or sustainably managed forests.

This project has been assisted by the Cochlear Implant Club and Advisory Association, the Royal Institute for Deaf and Blind Children, and Cochlear Limited.

Contents

**The basic attribute of mankind
is to look after each other.**

Ophthalmologist and humanitarian,
Fred Hollows AC (1929–93)

FOREWORD

The first time I had the pleasure of becoming acquainted with Professor Bill Gibson was during a cocktail party at Government House in 2003 to thank the donors of the Menière's Research Foundation. It was two years into my term as Governor of New South Wales and I had recently become the foundation's patron-in-chief. I was aware that Professor Gibson's two areas of expertise are cochlear implant surgery and Menière's disease, which affects a person's hearing and their balance. He demonstrated his passion for finding a cure for this debilitating condition during his talk and afterwards, as he mingled with guests, he revealed himself to be a warm, friendly man who has the ability to get on with people from all walks of life. I experienced first-hand his caring nature when he treated one of the guests who had succumbed to a dizzy spell and was then able to participate in the remainder of the evening.

There is a long tradition of caring among members of Bill Gibson's family, including his great-grandfather, grandfather and father, who were all doctors. Bill was born in Devon in 1944 while his father was at the D-Day landings in Normandy. Inspiration while growing up came from stories of his father's role as a 'medic' during World War II and also the general practice he ran from the family home. By the age of five Bill knew that he wanted to be a doctor. He gained a full scholarship to the Middlesex Hospital Medical School in London, where 'the best decision' he ever made was agreeing to a minor role in a hospital production of *A Man for All Seasons* because he met his future wife, Alex, when she made him up to look Spanish. Alex has been by his side ever since and provided support throughout his career.

Bill Gibson met some of the first doctors and scientists to become involved with the design and clinical use of the cochlear implant in the UK and the US. In 1983, he departed one of the top ENT consultant posts in the UK to emigrate with his family to Australia, where his identical twin brother was already living. Before leaving London, he attended a talk by Professor Graeme Clark, who said to him, 'I hope you'll work with me on the cochlear implant program in Australia'.

In his new professorial role at the University of Sydney and Royal Prince Alfred Hospital, Bill Gibson was one of the first surgeons to use the commercialised version of Professor Clark's bionic ear which is manufactured and distributed today by Cochlear Limited. The author of this biography, Tina Allen, uses her medical writing skills to explain how the bionic ear works and provides vignettes of more than forty of the adults and children he implanted with this device between 1984 and 2014.

Bill Gibson received harsh criticism when he started performing cochlear implant operations on children, particularly those born deaf. Some of the most strident opposition came from members of the Deaf community and also educational authorities of the day, who thought that deaf children should be taught Sign Language in special schools. He showed great wisdom and foresight when he progressively lowered the age of the children who received cochlear implants, because he knew that their brains would be more receptive to speech and language development at a younger age. Today, newborn babies in Australia have their hearing tested in hospital using the automated auditory brainstem response procedure he recommended to a ministerial committee. It is accepted clinical practice for babies found to be profoundly deaf to be assessed as candidates for a cochlear implant during the first year of life.

When I first met Bill Gibson, he was director of the Sydney Cochlear Implant Centre (SCIC) in Gladesville and today this charitable organisation has expanded into twelve centres around New South Wales and in Darwin. In 2013, when nearing the end of my term as Governor of New South Wales, I was invited to open the SCIC in Penrith, which caters for clients in the western suburbs of Sydney, the Blue Mountains and beyond. I was patron of the SCIC at that time and I witnessed the rapport Bill Gibson shares with his patients and also his sense of humour when he gave me a Hilaire Belloc poem about Lord Lundy, who was sent to govern New South Wales. It is important that we preserve for future generations the story of this pioneering cochlear implant surgeon who fought for hearing-impaired people everywhere to have equitable access to this remarkable medical innovation, regardless of their age, other disabilities or financial situation. Professor Bill Gibson is an outstanding man, a great humanitarian and deserving of this well-researched biography about his exceptional contribution to medicine.

Marie Bashir

Professor The Honourable
Dame Marie Bashir AD CVO

PREFACE

There can be few innovations in
medicine that have required so
much input from so many disciplines.

Professor Graeme Clark,
pioneer of the bionic ear

When Susan Walters was struck down at twenty-two years of age by a severe bout of meningococcal meningitis, she spent seven weeks recovering in hospital. Her sight returned and she learned to walk again, but her hearing stubbornly refused to return and she was declared 'stone deaf'. Susan's parents took her to a Sydney ear, nose and throat (ENT) surgeon who just happened to be looking for a candidate for a new device called the cochlear implant. They were a perfect fit. The surgery to restore Susan's hearing in August 1984 was not only a first for New South Wales, but for her surgeon, Professor Bill Gibson, as well.

This book is a celebration of the life and career of the pioneering ENT surgeon, Emeritus Professor Bill Gibson AO. On the eve of his retirement, this book also commemorates the thirty years he spent in the role of director of the Sydney Cochlear Implant Centre (SCIC). Between 1984 and 2014, Professor Gibson performed in excess of 2000 cochlear implant surgeries and became one of the most prolific surgeons in this field, yet few outside academic and clinical circles have heard of him. His great experience led to him modifying the surgical incision from a large C-shaped flap of skin to a small, straight incision behind the ear which has been adopted by surgeons around the world and greatly reduced the rate of wound breakdown.

Australians are leaders in the fields of sleep apnoea, ultrasound imaging and the cervical cancer vaccine, to name only a few, but one of our most successful medical innovations and exports is the multi-channel cochlear implant or 'bionic ear'. Designed by Professor Graeme Clark and his team of researchers and engineers in Melbourne, the bionic ear is sold today by Cochlear Limited in one-hundred countries and is used by more than 250 000 people. The development of this device in Melbourne has been well documented in biographies and other non-fiction books,[1] but the Sydney side of this story is less well known. Not only was Professor Clark's proto-type design commercialised in Sydney by Paul Trainor's Nucleus Group, but it was Bill Gibson, a Sydney surgeon, who contributed in a significant way to making the bionic ear a clinical success. It is a well-established principle that a new medical device requires clinical application or it will end up gathering dust on a shelf.

Professor Gibson operated on some of the very early patients to receive the commercialised version of the bionic ear, who were also some of the first to show outstanding speech recognition. Only six months after her cochlear implant operation at Royal Prince Alfred Hospital in Sydney, Susan Walters was filmed in a split-screen video talking on the telephone to Professor Gibson. He believes this to be the first demonstration anywhere in the world that a cochlear implant could deliver enough information for a recipient to under-stand speech without lip-reading or contextual clues. When he showed the filmed conversation at international conferences, American colleagues asked if they could talk with Sue on the phone themselves.

After successfully restoring the hearing of twenty adults with the bionic ear, Professor Gibson performed a cochlear implant operation on the first paediatric recipient in the world: four-year-old Holly

McDonell, who had been completely deafened by meningitis eight months earlier. Within seven months of her operation in June 1987, Holly was able to cope in a kindergarten glass of thirty pupils at a mainstream public school. A congenitally deaf girl who received a cochlear implant, Pia Jeffrey, featured on the front page of the *Sydney Morning Herald* when she heard her first sounds at six years of age and her photo would later appear on the back cover of the Sydney telephone directory. The stories of Susan Walters, Holly McDonell and Pia Jeffrey, as well as many other cochlear implant recipients, are documented in this biography.

Professor Gibson came under intense criticism when he began implanting progressively younger children and then finally babies. This was viewed by many as child abuse because the children couldn't consent to the procedure and educators thought they should be taught Sign Language. He received hate mail from those opposed to the new technology, even though it provided profoundly deaf children with the opportunity to sit next to their hearing peers in classrooms and aspire to the same goals in academia, sport and the visual arts.

After helping to make the bionic ear a success in Australia, in both adults and children, Professor Gibson continued to champion Professor Clark's bionic ear, demonstrating the intricate surgery in countries such as New Zealand, China, India and South America. He also trained dozens of young surgeons, who travelled to Australia from around the world to spend six months operating at his side. By generously sharing his knowledge, he has assisted countless hearing-impaired people from around the world while promoting a proudly Australian invention. Since their first devices rolled off the production line in 1982, Cochlear has continued production in Sydney and contributes millions of dollars to the Australia economy every year.

The walls of Professor Gibson's clinical rooms are decorated with his surgical qualifications, the Order of Australia and many other accolades, including one of the inaugural 'Hearo Awards' from Cochlear in 2008. His patients refer to him as 'the good Prof' or 'Professor Bill', but mostly just as 'Prof'.

In 2009, I was commissioned by the Cochlear Implant Club and Advisory Association (CICADA) to write Professor Gibson's biography. Members of this club told me about his dedication and his sense of humour, as well as his love of dressing up and keenness to socialise with his patients – traits not normally associated with a medical specialist. After this build-up, I was curious to discover if he was brilliant or boorish, a raconteur or an egomaniac. The only way to find out was to meet him, which was no easy task. Despite being in his mid-sixties, Professor Gibson still had a full schedule of surgeries, clinics and meetings.

Bill and Alex Gibson didn't need to tell me that they were from England – their rounded vowels gave them away as soon as they welcomed me into their townhouse in Sydney's inner west. Bill told me that for as long as he can remember he wanted to be a doctor like his father, grandfather, great-grandfather and other members of his extended family.

He has a rich heritage and readers can use the Gibson Family Tree to trace the family members mentioned in this biography back to his Irish great-grandparents, George and Laura (see the Gibson family tree, page xvii). For many who are the subject of a biography, their childhood can be summed up in a few paragraphs, or possibly a chapter, but I have deliberately panned the camera slowly over Bill Gibson's formative years, which occupy the first two chapters of this book.

Accounts of childhood adventures with his identical twin brother in Devon display his initiative and high spirits, while anecdotes about his medical career in London and Sydney suggest an absent-minded professor absorbed in his search for a cure for that most disorienting and debilitating of maladies, Menière's disease.

No one could have been a more willing or patient subject of a biography than Professor Gibson, who I take the liberty of referring to as Bill throughout this book – from his delightful childhood to his distinguished present.

Late in 2012, Professor Gibson retired from his chair at the University of Sydney, but he is not yet ready to retire altogether. He continues to see his patients at the SCIC in his role as the founding director. Here he cuts a distinguished, almost nautical, figure in his navy sports blazer with brass buttons. Other trademarks of his wardrobe include his bright yellow socks and ties adorned with snails, which are the symbol of the SCIC as *cochlea* is the Latin word for snail. The SCIC is currently the largest provider of cochlear implants in Australia and its dozen regional centres, in locations convenient for its clients, are a tangible legacy of his career.

I hope you enjoy this journey of discovery about the wonderful gift of hearing and the inspiring work of Professor Bill Gibson, who has dedicated his life to returning this vital sense to as many people as possible.

Tina Allen

ABBREVIATIONS

3M	Minnesota Mining and Manufacturing
AABR	automated auditory brainstem response
BACO	British Academic Conference in Otolaryngology
BPPV	benign paroxysmal positional vertigo
CCIC	Children's Cochlear Implant Centre
CICADA	Cochlear Implant Club and Advisory Association
CORLAS	Collegium Oto-Rhino-Laryngologicum Amicitiae Sacrum
EABR	electric auditory brainstem response
EAR Foundation	Ear and Allied Research Foundation
ECochG	electrocochleography
ENT	ear, nose and throat
FDA	Food and Drug Administration (US)
LION	Live International Otolaryngology Network
MB	Bachelor of Medicine
MD	Doctorate of Medicine
NHS	National Health Scheme
OAE	otoacoustic emissions
OLSA	Otolaryngology Association of Australia
PDSG	Profound Deafness Study Group
RCS	Royal College of Surgeons of England
RIDBC	Royal Institute of Deaf and Blind Children
RPA Hospital	Royal Prince Alfred Hospital
SCIC	Sydney Cochlear Implant Centre
SWISH	NSW Statewide Infant Screening – Hearing
TGA	Therapeutic Goods Administration
UCH	University College Hospital

GIBSON FAMILY TREE

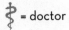 = doctor

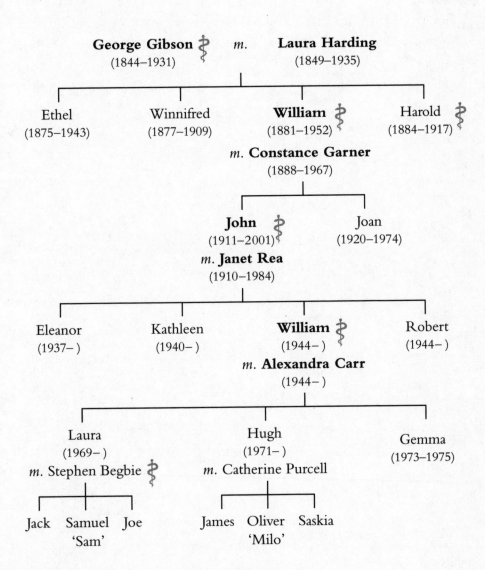

George Gibson *m.* **Laura Harding**
(1844–1931) (1849–1935)

Ethel
(1875–1943)

Winnifred
(1877–1909)

William
(1881–1952)
m. **Constance Garner**
(1888–1967)

Harold
(1884–1917)

John
(1911–2001)
m. **Janet Rea**
(1910–1984)

Joan
(1920–1974)

Eleanor
(1937–)

Kathleen
(1940–)

William
(1944–)
m. **Alexandra Carr**
(1944–)

Robert
(1944–)

Laura
(1969–)
m. Stephen Begbie

Hugh
(1971–)
m. Catherine Purcell

Gemma
(1973–1975)

Jack   Samuel   Joe
'Sam'

James   Oliver   Saskia
'Milo'

CHAPTER 1

Memories of a father at war

I heard the stories so often I took
them into me ... and now, mine or
not, they are my shiniest self.

Anna Funder, *All that I Am*

We are all born in the middle of something. For William Gibson and his twin brother Robert it just happened to be World War II. The twins were born on 11 June 1944 into a household of women in the county of Devonshire while their father was away in Normandy serving as a commanding officer for the D-Day landings. Captain John Gibson faced all the dangers of being on the front line, but he was not involved in the armed combat on the beaches or the landing grounds or the fields. His role with the Royal Army Medical Corps was far more inspirational in the eyes of his children, particularly one of his two sons, who would later become a doctor.

The boys' mother, Jane Gibson, knew she was having twins and telephoned Nurse Webb to come as soon as the labour pains started. A birthing room was no place for little girls so Jane's mother took Eleanor, aged seven, and Kathy, aged four, to spend the day with their auntie Nell. Jane and the elderly nurse ensconced themselves in one of the large upstairs bedrooms of Lakemead, in the old walled town of Totnes on the river Dart. The babies were born without complication at about 4 o'clock.

Eleanor remembers arriving home from her auntie Nell's with her sister and climbing up the carpeted stairs. 'We found our mother resting on a large bed with a tightly wrapped bundle on each side of her,' says Eleanor, who was informed that William was born before Robert and that Nurse Webb would be staying for their mother's lying-in.

That evening Jane composed a telegram for John, who was by now stationed at one of the Allied headquarters in the south of France. He had been away from them for long periods over the last four and half years since World War II began.

SEPTEMBER 1939

John and Jane Gibson were living in Birmingham when they heard the BBC announcement by the British Prime Minister, Neville Chamberlain, on 3 September 1939 that Britain had declared war on Germany. After John enlisted with the Royal Army Medical Corps, Jane took two-year-old Eleanor down to Totnes in Devon. Jane would have the company of her widowed mother, known affectionately as 'Ammy' by all her family.

Totnes also felt like home for Jane, who was the youngest of four children to be born in the headmaster's residence of the King Edward VI Grammar School. Her father, Charles Rea, who was appointed the first lay headmaster in 1896,[1] had enjoyed holidays touring the continent on a bicycle with a camera slung over his shoulder. The family thought these trips were opportunities to get away for a few months from Ammy, who was 'reputedly an awkward person' and also extremely religious.[2] This tiny, bespectacled woman asked the staff from the school to drag a piano onto the High Street, where she became a regular fixture on Sundays, playing hymns to encourage the townsfolk to go to church.

When Jane's brother Louis died from appendicitis at age nine in 1914, grief was the mostly likely reason her father Charles replaced his academic gowns with mayoral robes to serve three one-year terms as his contribution to World War I. He also spent many years transcribing the town's historical records and writing articles for the Totnes Antiquarian Society.[3] After the war, Jane's parents purchased a sandstone and slated house in Maudlin Road, Lakemead, on a hill overlooking Totnes. Only a decade after the Rea family moved into this home, Charles died of bowel cancer in March 1929.

Jane was only eighteen when she attended her father's grand funeral, which included a mayoral procession through the streets of Totnes, headed by the town crier and mace bearers.[4] Her mother Ammy never really came out of mourning and continued to wear dark dresses for the remaining three decades of her life. And so it was to her pious and widowed mother and the two remaining staff at Lakemead that a pregnant Jane took Eleanor to live during World War II.

With his family settled, Captain John Gibson reported for duty at the Aldershot Barracks in Hampshire, 40 miles south-west of London. In his account of the war[5] John wrote that he doubled as the sports officer while he 'saw in' the recruits through a three-month course in hygiene and first aid. When he was home on leave in Totnes John held the first of his war-time babies, Kathleen, who was named for her strong Irish heritage. Kathy, as she became known, was born in 1940, the same year that the Battle of Britain began. During air raids Jane grabbed Kathy from her cot and ran down two flights of stairs to the basement, where the Luftwaffe provided her lullaby and the family huddled under blankets with the cook and the gardener.

After two years of looking after the health and fitness of his men in first Hampshire and then the Alva Valley in Scotland, John told Jane he would soon be seeing some action. The 'phoney war', as he called the previous period of limbo, was finally over. Into the top pocket of his khaki-coloured woollen uniform John buttoned a small black-and-white photo of Jane which did not do justice to her natural beauty.

John's ship was the first in the fleet to land on the African coast on 8 November 1942 and he made note of the 'twinkling lights of Algiers' to their left. In the northern Tunisian town of Medjes-el-Bab, John and his six orderlies set up a field ambulance station in a farmhouse with a red 'X' painted on the roof. The only access road to this farmhouse was frequently shelled by Germans, who occupied the hills surrounding the town.

Jane would have been desperate for news from the front and John's whereabouts, but all she received back in Devon were pale-yellow, index-sized cards bearing the name 'John Gibson', with ticks in boxes corresponding to his physical condition. She never really knew where he was.

After serving three months in North Africa, John's division arrived at the Mersey Docks in Liverpool and he was sent back up to Scotland. When he was granted fourteen days' leave, he returned to his family in Totnes, and his twin sons were born nine months later.

During the early months of 1944, John was stationed 200 miles east of Totnes in Newhaven, where he was assigned a trusted position on the planning team for the invasion of France. In the evenings he collected all the 'bumph' from Planning and worked till early in the morning organising the supplies to be loaded onto various ships.

In April 1944, John returned to Totnes when Jane was in the seventh month of her pregnancy. He looks tall in a photo taken of him in uniform during this brief leave. The diminutive Jane was only a week away from her delivery date when John departed from Newhaven for Operation Overlord, which history would remember as the D-Day landings.

John Gibson and his men from the Third Infantry Division set off at midnight on 5 June 1944. He recalled that dawn was a 'wonderful', though noisy, sight with assault craft numbering at least 3000 stretching as far as he could see. HMS *Warspite* fired its 15-inch guns across them and Royal Air Force planes flew over them like great freight trains rattling the sky. As Sword Beach came into view, a mortar hit the front ramp of John's landing craft, leaving it gaping and vulnerable.

Among those John knew from the landing party who waded ashore at 0700 were Craven and Watty, along with the war artist John Ward. John remained on the craft to treat the wounded and by the time he had transferred the last of them to a support vessel it was 0830. The beaches were 'not healthy' so John found his orderly and batman as quickly as possible and together they advanced westward the 20 miles through the French countryside to their headquarters in a château at Colleville-sur-Mer. That evening John's thoughts turned to his great friends Watty and Craven, who never made it off Sword Beach.

Nineteen days after D-Day, near a crossroads about a mile from the HQ, the division padre walked towards John holding a dog-eared telegram which announced the birth of his twin sons. John looked up and thanked the Padre, who replied, *'Pas du tout'*. John heard this French phrase for 'Not at all' as 'Pa of two' and laughed out loud with joy and relief. The English padre also seemed to enjoy the double meaning of his little joke.

For the first month at least after D-Day John remained at Colleville-sur-Mer as commander of the field ambulance station.

He used his limited knowledge of French to convince the countess who owned the château to allow his men to use her cellar so they had somewhere private to write their letters home. John Ward, whose art works were later acquired by the Imperial War Museum in London, used pen and paper to capture these poignant moments in the cellar. When Jane sent across a photo of herself with Bill and Bob, this same war artist remarked to John, 'Your wife looks well; the lights are back in her hair'.

The servicemen John treated had ailments ranging from gunshot wounds to battle exhaustion to ruptured eardrums, for which he was able to give penicillin for the first time in his career. It was not until World War II that large-scale production of penicillin commenced in America, allowing its more widespread use.

In August 1944 John and his men left Colleville-sur-Mer as part of a convoy of trucks, which zigzagged in a roughly eastward direction along rutted brown roads through French hedgerow country. When they reached the town of Flers, John found a little terrier which he named Joe Flers. This dog was run over by a tank but it must have made an impression on John because he later bought a similar breed for his children. The division stopped for a night near Rouen, where John bought a large bottle of Chanel No. 5 perfume for Jane. In Brussels they were met by cheering crowds, but by December John was spending a 'most uncomfortable and dodgy Christmas' by the river Maas in Holland. Lying in a ditch half-filled with snow and slush, John tried to keep warm in his camouflaged 'airborne' sleeping bag but never really felt safe because German air patrols came over every night.

The enemy encounters John faced as a medical officer with the Royal Army Medical Corps would later become burnished memories for his children, made brighter and more lustrous with each retelling. Bill has always been very proud of his father's role as a 'medic' during World War II and can recount several of his war-time stories in such animated detail they could easily have been his own. Among his favourites was the time his father needed to deliver drugs and dressings to a small hospital staffed by Germans, who were pleased to see him. When he arrived back to his division John discovered that he had accidentally crossed over into enemy territory. He wrote of this incident, 'I was greeted as a hero when I called again and didn't admit it was just bad map reading.'

Early in 1945 John had the harrowing task of liberating prisoners from a concentration camp. Then, in the days before Germany's surrender on 7 May 1945, he spent a night arranging ambulances on either side of a river in the process of being bridged so they could cross. 'We knew VE [Victory in Europe] Day was in the offing and I was scared stiff that my luck wouldn't hold out.'

With their bands and banners, 'a great gathering of the Devon clans' led a flickering torchlight procession down the High Street of Totnes on 8 May 1945 to honour those who had died.[6] John also celebrated VE Day with a parade of massed bands, but he was in Bremerhaven, a German seaport on the North Sea. Doctors were not demobbed until after the end of the war so they could repatriate the prisoners or wounded, if fit to travel, back to their own countries.

John was now a major and from Bremerhaven he moved to Luneburg Heath near Hamburg, where he worked shifts with another country doctor, Captain Jimmie Wells, from Oxfordshire. John had just gone off duty when the Allies apprehended one of the creators of the Holocaust, the Reichsführer (leader) of the SS, Heinrich Himmler. While being examined by Captain Wells, Himmler crunched down on a tiny glass vial of cyanide, which he had concealed in a fold of his cheek, and died within minutes.[7] John wrote of this moment, which has been documented by war historians: 'The other [Medical Officer] was most unfairly criticized for missing this, for I'm sure I would have missed it too.'

* * *

Soon after the war officially ended in September 1945, John Gibson arrived at Lakemead in a grey pinstripe suit, having given his Army uniform away. Among the trophies of war he brought home were a pair of Zeiss binoculars and a silver cigarette case, which held the little vials of heroin and adrenalin he administered on the battlefield.

Bill and Bob had never met their father, so this new playfellow was a pleasant distraction, but it was a different matter for their sisters, for whom he was like a stranger. John had missed many of his children's formative years and found it difficult to show the affection he felt for them – 'perhaps too great an affection', as he noted in his account of the war.

John had not completed his clinical training before the war began so for six months he delivered babies at Oldway, a mock-Versailles mansion near Paignton owned by the Singer family of sewing machine fame. He then worked for a further six months in the exclusive coastal resort town of Torquay at the Torbay Hospital.

On his rare days off John took his family on expeditions around Totnes. Once they reached the High Street it was only a short stroll along the covered Butterwalk to the Guildhall. For the Gibson children this town hall was not only a history lesson but a lesson in family history. There are large oak tables on the first floor where Oliver Cromwell sat with Lord Fairfax in 1646 to plan the civil wars, and also a portrait gallery, which includes ancestors from both the maternal and paternal sides of Bill's family who had served terms as mayor of the Borough – including a grandfather and his two great-grandfathers.

Near the Guildhall are the remains of one of the earliest Norman strongholds, Totnes Castle. Looking north from the castle ramparts on a clear day it is possible to see all the way to the Dartmoor nature park, with its deserted miles of tor and bog which range in colour from moss green to rust brown. Jane and John took photos of each other on Dartmoor holding the handle of a large nanny-style pram. Sitting upright inside are a pair of rosy-cheeked, white-blonde toddlers, Bill and Bob, and holding onto each side of the pram are their sisters, Eleanor and Kathy.

On their return from these day trips, the family entertained themselves in the sitting room of Lakemead, reading stories and listening to Ammy playing pieces such as Beethoven's *Moonlight Sonata* on her grand piano. For Bill and his siblings, this sonata still evokes memories of their grandmother, as does the plodding dum-dum-de-dum of Chopin's *Funeral March*, which Ammy played at all hours of the night and day on the second grand piano in her late husband's study.

To the Gibson children their grandmother's garden of an acre and a half seemed enormous. If they walked across the level lawn from the sitting room there was a swing hanging from the branches of an ancient cedar tree. The remainder of the garden fell steeply away from this cedar and at the bottom of the grass banks there was a fragrant rose garden where the children searched for Saxon silver pennies. Like the Old Town walls, which had once protected the early Saxon settlers and their mint, the stone walls of this garden made the Gibson children feel safe. With its brick stables, tennis lawn and heated glasshouse for the grapevines, the property was like a little village, but how long would they remain living here now that the war was over and their father had returned home?

It wasn't only their mother who loved the fruitful South Hams district; it also had a very special place in their father's heart. As a young lad John travelled down from the industrial city of Birmingham in the West Midlands to spend his school holidays, and also much of World War I, with his grandparents in Devon.

George and Laura Gibson lived at 13 Bridgetown Road, in an exclusive suburb on the eastern side of the river Dart in Totnes. They employed a staff of six to run their Victorian home, St Maur, including a boy to run the medicines for George's medical practice. They were used to having a large staff from the eighteen years George served as a Colonel-Surgeon with the British Army until his retirement in 1888. While living in Totnes he served terms as both mayor and medical officer of health.

John was an only child until his sister, Joan, came along when he was nine, so he enjoyed playing with his cousins during these holidays with his grandparents in Totnes. George owned some of the first cars in Devon, including a 1925 Bean, a Model T Ford and a Wolseley, which he permitted John to drive from the age of about eleven onwards.

When John was seventeen and on holidays in Totnes from boarding at Epsom College in Surrey, he noticed a girl in a black dress standing next to the bridge over the river Dart. She was selling cornflowers, which, like poppies, were sold as symbols of Remembrance Day because both continued to grow on the barren battlefields after World War I. The girl's name was Janet but she said to him, 'You can call me Jane'. She was in mourning for her beloved father, Charles Rea, the day that John bought a cornflower from her and it became their own remembrance flower thereafter.

There would only be one woman in John's life. After a seven-year courtship, protracted mainly by his medical studies, he married Jane Rea in 1935 in the 15th-century St Mary's in Totnes, which has a lofty bell tower at one end. One of the eight bells in this tower had been recast and donated by Jane's grandfather, Thomas Kellock, who founded the legal practice in the High Street of Totnes (which continued until 2016) and served four terms as mayor of the borough between 1865 and 1896. Other ceremonies that took place in this church were the grand funeral of Jane's Irish father, Charles Rea, and the baptism of her twin sons, William Peter Rea Gibson and Robert John Rea Gibson, who received a common middle name in memory of the grandfather they never met.

For the first dozen years of their married life John and Jane had endured long absences from each other and always lived with family, first in Birmingham with John's parents and then in Totnes with Jane's mother, Ammy. John's first priority was to find a suitable dwelling for his family and a position for himself nearby, but Britain was cash-strapped after the war and jobs were in extremely short supply.

In March 1946 John applied for the position of practice assistant for Bob Sammons in the seaside resort of Dawlish. There were 150 applicants but fortunately John had excellent references from the Torbay Hospital and was successful in securing the position. He remained close friends with his replacement at the hospital, Roger Blackney, with whom he played squash on a weekly basis for the next twenty years. Within six months John could afford to buy a one-third share in Bob Sammons's practice and a home in Dawlish.

The family took up residence in their new home in December 1946 as the first snow began to fall. By late January 1947 there was an almost unprecedented white-out across Devon that lasted until mid-March. This didn't worry the Gibson family. John expresses their feelings so well in the closing line of his account of the war: '[We had] no money, no furniture, but how happy we were ...'

* * *

The four Gibson children would all come to prefer Dawlish, the seaside town with its mild climate and subtropical plants, to Totnes, the upland town. Situated on a bejewelled stretch of coastline known as the Devon Riviera, Dawlish has provided inspiration for novelists such as Jane Austen and Charles Dickens, who both made visits in the early 1800s. The town was also popular with royalty and the gentry, who came for the summer season complete with servants and friends.

It was not only for the sea-bathing and brightly coloured changing huts that visitors have travelled to Dawlish for the last three centuries. There are also the clear, trout-filled waters of 'The Brook', which flows through the town centre towards the sea under a series of decorative stone bridges, and the unique position of the railway line. Designed by Isambard Kingdom Brunel, the line follows the curves of the Devon coastline from Dawlish to Plymouth so closely that waves regularly wash over the railway carriages.

Heading eastwards from the Dawlish railway station, where the main road to Exeter veers sharply away from the sea, there is a street on the left called East Cliff Road. The Gibson family's new home was halfway up this road's steep incline, past a series of substantial houses with well-stocked gardens. Its imposing entrance posts display the name Whickham Lodge and are flanked by dry-stone entrance walls with rings where horses could be tethered. One of Bill's earliest aural memories of this home was the 'clip clop' of Mr Tapper's horse, which pulled the cart loaded with coke for his family's boiler and the coal for the their fireplaces.

Whickham Lodge had bells which former inhabitants would have used to summon servants to the four bedrooms at the front of the house overlooking the sea, including the room shared by Bill and his brother. There was also accommodation for two servants accessed by a separate staircase leading up from the back kitchen, scullery and cellar. A lodger named Fred Lloyd occupied one of these rooms and his board would have contributed to Jane's housekeeping money.

The lofty, echoing rooms were soon partially filled with pieces from Totnes, including one of Ammy's prized grand pianos, and a grandfather clock from Bill's paternal grandparents in Birmingham. Bill remembers his mother writing her letters at a Victorian ladies' desk near the dining room and taking the telephone calls for his father's surgery in the kitchen. 'Mum was very homely and hardworking,' says Bill of his mother, who did all the housework and gardening as well as running his father's medical practice.

On weekends and bank holidays, Bill explored local attractions with his family but every second Sunday they returned to Totnes to have lunch with Ammy. He recalls that when his family first moved to Dawlish they all needed to fit into his father's Austin A70, which had no seat belts. 'Usually Bob and I would sit with Dad on the front bench seat while Mum and the girls sat on the back seat. If Dad had to stop suddenly he would put his left arm out to stop us going through the windscreen. There were teeth marks in the dashboard so we were lucky we didn't break our necks.'

During the 16-mile trip from Dawlish to Totnes, John had to stop at the same field nearly every time for Bill and Bob to vomit. One of Jane's tricks to help prevent the boys from becoming bored and carsick was reciting in her best Devonshire accent the verses of a traditional song about a fair on the western edge of Dartmoor, 'Goosey Fair':

> And it's oh, and where be a-going,
> And what be a-doing of there,
> Heave down your prong and stamp along,
> To Tavistock Goosey Fair.

At one of these Sunday lunches Ammy most likely expressed horror at Jane looking after Whickham Lodge on her own, because a suitable young woman from Dawlish was soon found to help her, three half-days a week. Margie, who was about eighteen when she started, also babysat Bill and his brother when their parents went out at night. John and Jane enjoyed evening functions at the local golf club, which were a good opportunity for people to meet the new doctor in town.

The entrance to John's surgery was further down the driveway side of Whickham Lodge to the entrance used by the family. It comprised a waiting room, a surgery for patient consultations and a small room in between where John examined patients and performed simple pathology tests using the reagents and small brass microscope on the shelf. Bill was not permitted into these rooms during surgery hours and the first time he saw his father examining a patient was at the Dawlish Cottage Hospital at Christmas, when it was looking festive with decorations.

Bill's father took it in turns to do the Christmas rounds at the Cottage Hospital with the three other doctors in Dawlish: Bob Sammons, Alec Lees and Douglas Peterkin. The biggest change for these general practitioners was the introduction in 1948 of the National Health Service (NHS) by Aneurin Bevan, the Secretary of State for Health in Attlee's post-war Labour government. Bill's father told him that 'Bevan initially bribed the NHS consultant surgeons with gold, but after a while their pay didn't seem so much and they started to feel diddled'.

Patients no longer had to pay for their medical visits, but Bill remembers many of them expressing their gratitude by giving his father pots of Devonshire cream, eggs, butter and other farm produce. This was a great help for his mother as food rationing was still in place in the United Kingdom until 1954. Fortunately, Jane was a good cook. Rice puddings and steak and kidney pies were family favourites but it was the burnt toffee aromas from her treacle tarts that brought Bill running to the kitchen. The children also contributed to the larder by collecting mussels from the pebbly coves near the Main Beach of Dawlish, which their mother transformed into an array of tasty dishes, including curries.

A fair bit of bartering went on between the townsfolk and the medical professionals also helped each other out from time to time. One of John Gibson's more unusual requests was to attend the surgery of Dougy Knight, the dentist in Dawlish, to administer anaesthetics for his patients. Dougy was a family friend so John did not mind performing this service but Bill says, 'It would be frowned upon today because if the patient vomited in the dentist's chair they could choke.'

Medical practices were very different from the present day. John Gibson conducted a drop-in surgery from nine until ten in the morning and from six until seven in the evening, but in reality patients rang the doorbell and pounded on his surgery door at any time of the day or evening. The children were not allowed to play rambunctious games during surgery hours so Jane needed to do a lot of 'shushing' when the girls were not at St Margaret's School in Exeter and the boys were not at the local kindergarten.

The twins were not only identical in appearance but would speak as a pair, saying things such as '*Our* father is in the surgery' or 'Can *we* have a sweet?' This pattern of communication was established early because Bill assumed the role of the older brother (albeit by ten minutes) and often answered on his brother's behalf. If, for instance, their father asked Bob if he wanted more pudding, Bill instinctively replied for him, 'No, he doesn't'.

While the boys were undoubtedly amusing, they could also be mischievous. The night their sister Eleanor felt caterpillars squirming in her pyjamas and bedclothes John could be heard shouting, 'Mother, deal with the twins!' This usually meant being sent to their room because Eleanor cannot remember their mother 'ever laying a finger on the boys'.

'If one of us got into trouble,' says Bill, 'both of us got the blame. Even mum couldn't tell us apart if we were down the garden, so sometimes she called out "Billybob!"'

As the sons of the local GP, Bill says they were 'marked'. When patients noticed two very blond boys around town, reports of their antics arrived home before they did. The time they mounted the horn of a Model T Ford on the handlebars of their bike and startled some old ladies with their honking in a Dawlish back alley, John could again be heard calling from his surgery, 'Mother – the twins!'

There was an assortment of pets at Whickham Lodge, including a budgie, a goldfish and a white cat with blue eyes named Daisy, who was deaf but had a long life. Bill also remembers a Jack Russell with a wiry, white coat of hair. Their father named this little dog Joe, after the one he'd found in the French city of Flers during the war, but it was naughty and stole the patients' belongings. 'Joe lasted about a year,' says Bill. 'Then Dad sent him back to the farm – or at least that's where we were told he went.'

When Bill saw the muscles of a dog continue to twitch after it had been run over by a car, he asked his father, 'Why did it keep moving?' John told him, 'It's because of his nerves.' This reply must have raised as many questions for Bill as it did answers, because from the age of about five he knew he wanted to be a doctor. He says, 'It never crossed my mind that I would do anything else'.

CHAPTER 2

Bill's school days

Dad was pleased that I did
well academically and he forgave
me my lack of sporting prowess.

Bill Gibson

B ill spent the first six 'very happy' years of his school life with his
brother in a two-storey Victorian schoolhouse, which was
smothered in dark-green ivy. The upstairs windows of Beacon
School afforded the preparatory school boys a glorious view of the
coastline near the village of Teignmouth (pronounced 'tinmuth'),
which was a bus trip of three miles along the coast road from
Dawlish. At the front door of the schoolhouse there was a set of out-
wardly curving steps where the sixty or so boys in their grey blazers,
trimmed in bottle green, lined up each year for the school photo.
Seated in the middle of this photo were the headmaster and his wife,
Mr and Mrs Daunt.

Bill and his brother arrived in 1950, when Beacon School was
still very much 'a family affair', because the Daunts lived with their
two children, Timothy and Jenifer, in a private section of the
schoolhouse. During maths and French lessons, with Mr Hadley and

Mr Topham respectively, Bill could hear the far-off yapping of the Daunts' corgis, Yargi and Jasper, and the crunch of Margery Daunt's pumps as she walked along the gravel driveway, with a clutch of bantam chicks chirping brightly as they followed behind her.

For history lessons, Leslie Daunt pulled a world map down from the wall and told the boys that the deep pink parts represented the British Empire, but in reality, the map was steadily losing its rosiness. Bill recalls that India had already gained its 'bloody' independence and the Suez Crisis in Egypt would erupt during his last year at Beacon School. The balding Mr Daunt with his rimless glasses was a graduate of Trinity College, Oxford, and inspired in Bill a lifelong love of history. He named the school houses after three famous Elizabethans and placed the twins in the house named after Sir Walter Raleigh – the dashing Devonshire-born soldier who reputedly laid down his cloak over a puddle for Queen Elizabeth I.

Sir Walter Raleigh was one of the famous Brits who featured in the vast Dome of Discovery which had been purpose built on the South Bank of the Thames for the 1951 Festival of Britain. It was quite an expedition to take a family of six to London but Bill's father considered it to be an educational experience for them all. Bill can remember a huge revolving drum, mounted on a wall, from which he and Bob came out vomiting, but it was the Big Dipper that topped the list of amusements for the pair of them. 'There was even a newsreel taken of Bob and me screaming as we were going down. If you see two little boys at the front looking terrified, that was us.'

The family also went to see the London Zoo, because the twins wanted to see the elephants and lions. Bill liked a poem about a lion in a zoo from a collection entitled *Cautionary Tales* by Hilaire Belloc. He can still recite today the poem 'Jim', about a boy who hadn't gone a yard away from his nanny at the zoo when:

With open Jaws, a lion sprang,
And hungrily began to eat
The Boy: beginning at his feet.
Now, just imagine how it feels
When first your toes and then your heels,
And then by gradual degrees,
Your shins and ankles, calves and knees,
Are slowly eaten, bit by bit.

After the Festival of Britain, the Gibson family ventured north the 120 miles from London to Birmingham to visit Bill's paternal grandparents, William and Constance. Con, as everyone called her, was very tall and beautiful. She walked gracefully and strove to maintain this poise for the rest of her life.[1] She told Bill that when she was seventeen she was part of a group who modelled outfits for Queen Alexandra at Buckingham Palace. Con's former occupation as a 'costume model' was most likely one of the reasons her wealthy parents-in-law in Totnes, George and Laura Gibson, didn't approve of her.

Con and William lived in two terrace houses which had been 'knocked together', at 10 Nechelles Park Road in a slum area of Birmingham. In his ground-floor surgery, Grandpa Gibson had an old wooden medicine cabinet mounted on the wall and he sat on an antique hooped chair which Bill says was 'designed to accommodate ladies' full skirts and petticoats'. William Gibson, who usually wore a three-piece suit and watch chain, was the last in a long line of family members to have been born in Ireland and these two items of furniture came from Cork.

Bill says that details about his Irish ancestry are 'a bit sketchy' but he knows that in about 1600 three Huguenot brothers left France to settle in Tipperary and start a woollen mill. It is thought that the brother's surname in France was Lechat and this was changed to

Gibbe, supposedly the Old Irish for cat, then later to Gibson.[2] Many of the family members could jump well, like cats, including William, who was the long-jumping champion at the London Hospital in 1903. Before settling in Birmingham, William had been a medical officer in World War I. He hated his war service because he had left behind his younger brother Harold in the cemetery in Calais, after he died in 1917 from gunshot wounds, received while treating the wounded.

On their return home from this trip to Birmingham Bill's father told him that Grandpa Gibson had prostate cancer, which 'he didn't like to talk about because he couldn't face the chemo'. Bill learned very early in life that prostate cancer is like the Sword of Damocles which hangs over a man's head by a thread. 'Even if it never actually falls,' Bill says, 'it signifies the impending doom of it happening.'

It transpired soon after his death that William was hopeless with money and had left Con with only a small estate. 'He was a general practitioner but half of his patients he never charged,' says Bill, who adds that his grandfather also gambled 'a fair bit'. Bill's grandmother would now be dividing her time between their home in Dawlish and the home of Bill's auntie Joan, his father's sister, who lived in New Maldon, on the southern outskirts of London. What Bill remembers most vividly from Con's extended stays in Dawlish were her ghost stories. 'Con told us that if we got out of bed during the night, a corpse would grab our ankles.'

During one of Con's visits, Bill and his brother conducted a trial run of the billy cart they had constructed from old pram parts. Their plan was to speed down the steep decline of East Cliff Road and veer sharply into one of the driveway entrances before they reached Exeter Road. 'All was going well until we saw Con standing in the last possible driveway we could turn into,' says Bill, who ran home and called out in unison with his brother, 'Con's down!' This was sufficient to communicate to their mother the calamitous news that they had felled their statuesque grandmother in one swoop.

Whatever punishment Bill and Bob received did not seem to deter them from further escapades. After a father-and-son discussion about why women wear 'stinky perfume', the twins considered they were 'doing their mother a favour' when they went up to their parents' room and emptied the contents of the large bottle of Chanel No. 5 into a sink in the corner of the room. Their mother was upset because it was the perfume their father had brought back for her from France after World War II.

* * *

When Bill and Bob were around ten years old their father decided they should learn how to safely handle and fire a gun, in case there was another war. He set up a target in the front garden of Whickham Lodge, near the cherry tree, and instructed them in the use of air guns with metal pellets. However, he never let the boys use a shot-gun and even showed them a patient with a gunshot wound as a deterrent.

Visits to army disposal stores with his father were always interesting for Bill because they sold the components of surplus aeroplanes from World War II. John paid about 50 shillings for a T1154 transmitter and companion receiver which Bill was given as a Christmas present so he could construct radios. Inspiration for this new hobby had come from a visit to Totnes where Bill discovered in Grandfather Rea's study an aerial linked to an early radio, which he describes as 'a lovely old thing'. Bill and Bob learnt to build crystal radios from scratch using a thimble, with a screw in the bottom, which they filled with solder. The radio was named for the crystal, which they then placed on top of the solder. By jiggling a little wire, called the 'cat's whisker', the twins could pick up the home services of the BBC and also Radio Luxembourg, which they preferred because it broadcast more popular music, such as Bill Haley & His Comets.

For a school project Bill made a one-valve set but the teachers disqualified him because they thought he must have had help from an adult or parent. He hadn't. Bill remembers another day when he and his classmates were told to wait outside the English master's office until their names were called. 'Bob told me he hadn't learnt the poem so I went in and did it for myself and then ten boys later I went in and recited it for my brother. He got a better mark.'

The determined way Bill set about each task was a character trait that would stand him in good stead in his quest to become a doctor. When he had done well in a set of exams, Leslie Daunt moved him up one school year. The year or two Bill spent in this class placed him at an advantage with the curriculum over Bob for the Common Entrance exam, which they sat together with the other twelve-year-olds in a hall at Beacon School.

The families had to indicate before this exam their choices of senior schools. Epsom College was selected as the first choice for the twins because their grandfather William and their father John had both attended the school. John was desperate for his sons to follow in his footsteps and this college prepared students for a medical career. A high mark was required for admission. The results were released in July and only Bill was offered a place. His parents decided he should remain at Beacon School with Bob until the end of 1956 while they explored their options. Over the coming months, Bill went through the motions of school and family life but the worry of not being sent to the same school as his brother weighed heavily on him.

During August the population of Dawlish doubled or even tripled and Bill's father ran a summer surgery from a rented house near the camping grounds of Dawlish Warren; a suburb situated on an elongated peninsula which extends out from the township of Dawlish into the river Exe estuary. Bill remembers this surgery being a lucrative part of his father's practice because the visitors needed pain relief for their sunburn or a fishhook through their finger or 'something else that was silly'.

Each September, right at the end of the school holidays, John employed a locum so the family could take a holiday to the north-west of Cornwall. They hired a caravan and camped in Trebetherick on a farmer's plot of land. This was halfway between the St Enodoc golf course and the surf beach at Polzeath, where Bill remembers bodysurfing on plywood boards. 'God, it was cold! But we only had one holiday each year and we were happy by the sea.'

Another annual family event Bill enjoyed was celebrating Guy Fawkes Day on 5 November. During the afternoon, Bill and his brother helped their father to build a bonfire, strategically placing potatoes wrapped in tinfoil so they could easily be retrieved later on. The fire drew all the family outside, where they assembled in a circle, palms turned towards to the warmth, faces bright with anticipation for the whoosh of the rockets, the fizz of the crackers and the whizz of the pinwheels nailed to a nearby wooden fence.

In December, as the school term drew to a close, Bill's parents confirmed his worst fears when they told him that he would be going to Epsom College on his own. 'That was when the migraines started,' says Bill. At first his father was not very sympathetic but later he asked his practice partner to examine Bill. 'Dr Sammons offered to do a lumbar puncture, but in the end he decided that I just didn't want to go to boarding school.' But the migraines – or 'mee-grains', as Bill calls them – were real.

On Christmas Day Bill attended St Gregory's church with his family, and afterwards there were usually about a dozen of his extended family members around the table for his mother's delicious roast turkey dinner. Taking pride of place in the middle of the table was a model which Bill's father had made in the days leading up to Christmas. 'Every year Dad made a little house from something like a shoebox. When we lifted the lid of the box, there were funny little presents inside, sitting on cotton wool.'

Bob returned to Beacon School in the New Year and remembers this parting as 'the beginning of me and Bill taking different paths'. For the twins their daily, even hourly, communion would be replaced by a distance of 200 miles when Bill became a boarder at Epsom College on the southern outskirts of London. Jane helped Bill to pack his huge trunk, including the shiny brass key ring engraved with his name and school number '317' which would hold his tuckbox and locker keys. 'Instead of keeping us together,' says Bill, with a wavering voice, 'we were separated. That was the saddest thing for me.'

* * *

In the first week of January 1957 Bill found himself travelling eastwards in his father's Austin towards Epsom Downs. John Gibson was very proud that his A70 could maintain a speed of 60 miles an hour, but each mile took Bill further away from wild and misty Devon, where seagulls screamed at the wind and fishing boats rocked rhythmically on their moorings. On their arrival at Epsom College Bill tried to keep up with his father's brisk pace as they walked towards the Carr boarding house near the main quadrangle. Being an old Epsonian, John knew his way to this boarding house, just as he knew all these gothic revival buildings with their slated turrets, stone bay windows and ecclesiastical flourishes.

Usually there were about a dozen new boys lined up outside the housemaster's office but Bill was the only one because the other first formers had all started the previous September, in the Michaelmas term. A second disadvantage Bill faced, which he thinks made him 'an easy target', was his feeling of insecurity at being separated from Bob. Within weeks of arriving he was caught chatting after lights out to another boy in the dormitory, Robert Dyke. A senior boy ordered Bill to the huge shared bathroom, where he gave him 'six with a slipper'. Bill also remembers the older boys hiding the knives and forks so the junior boys had no way of eating their food.

'Tom Brownish' is how Bill describes Epsom College and its boarding houses, because they remind him of Thomas Hughes's account of school life at Rugby School in *Tom Brown's School Days*. With its compulsory games, its insistence on good form and team spirit, its system of prefects and fagging, Epsom College was another typical English public school. Fagging involved juniors running errands and doing chores for the seniors. Bill recalls, 'You had to make toast for your prefect, you had to wash up their coffee mug and you had to clean their cadet's uniform'.

On the junior side of the Carr House dayroom, there was a large centrally placed table for the first formers to do their homework. In time Bill progressed to a 'toyce', which he describes as 'a little desk against the wall, with dividers between the desks where you could pin your own pictures'. On the senior side of the dayroom there was an ancient stag's head, complete with branching antlers, mounted on the wall, and cup-shaped sporting trophies of varying sizes arranged along the top of the dark wooden toyces.[3]

Epsom was unique among the public schools for holding athletics during the coldest months of the year, when the long jump pit was often frozen and white breath escaped from the mouths of boys as they exerted themselves. The appearance of snowbells alongside the waterlogged cross-country track in late January offered the first hope of spring, while Bill remembers the call of the cuckoo signalling its arrival.

The Lent term concluded at Easter, when Bill could go home for a few weeks, but the longest holiday of the year was at the conclusion of the summer term. From Paddington Station, Bill snoozed as he traversed the green fields of Berkshire and crisscrossed the Avon

Canal, waking in time for the conductor's whistle at St David's Station in Exeter. After changing trains, it was not long on Brunel's coast-hugging railway before he alighted at Dawlish.

There are four coves in Dawlish: Main Beach, Coryton Cove, Boat Cove and Shell Cove, where Bill and his brother enjoyed camping trips and scrambling over the rocks to collect mussels. Later on the twins worked out that they could wade around to Shell Cove at low tide, but when they were about thirteen they used to run through the Kennaway railway tunnel, which had been dug from the soft red sandstone of the seaside cliffs. When a train was coming, Bill and his brother had to lie down flat because there wasn't much room. As soon as they could see light again at each end of the tunnel, they breathed a collective sigh of relief and emerged at the other end with sooty faces.

The wild moorland of Dartmoor National Park was another favourite destination during the school holidays. Bill particularly enjoyed being taken by his father to a pub at Grimspound called The Warren. According to local folklore the fire in this pub had been burning for four or five hundred years and on one visit Bill wondered aloud what would happen if someone threw their beer on it. An old 'Dartymoor' fellow said in a reverent tone, 'It won't be gwain out if yer do that. It's been lit too long.' John told Bill and Bob more about World War II and they particularly enjoyed the stories about the D-Day landings and the telegram announcing their birth. John told them that he and Jane had chosen the names Elizabeth and Margaret in case they were girls. This amused Bill because he and Bob might have ended up with the same names as the Queen and her sister.

There was something about the Epsom Downs racetrack that reminds Bill of Royal Randwick (a turf club in Sydney). The boys from Epsom College were not permitted to attend the Epsom Derby, which is one of the highlights of the English horse racing season, but Bill enjoyed going for runs around the great expanse of open grassland adjacent to the racetrack and the college.

When he wasn't running or playing tennis, another of Bill's favourite pastimes was playing squash. During a game against his friend Robert Dyke, Bill was stung on his finger by a bee and his arm blew up like 'the Michelin Man'. Bill was given a shot of adrenalin at the Epsom General Hospital and then lay in the college sanatorium for three days, where the nursing sisters were very kind and gave him 'all this food'.

Bill had been best friends with Robert since his earliest days in Carr House and the 'slipper incident'. They had both been assigned to the D class, which was the least academically brilliant of the four classes, so it was a surprise when Bill came easily top of the form for physics in his O-levels. For English he came first in his form and second among all the students sitting the exam in the vicinity of Epsom, Surrey. This was undoubtedly assisted by the fact that he knew the whole of Shakespeare's play *Julius Caesar* by heart.

Despite Bill's success in physics and English, nothing could compensate for failing chemistry. At least half of the students in Bill's year wanted to do medicine so there were two medically oriented classes. Bill was told he would be put in the lower of these classes, Med Six B, which placed him at a distinct disadvantage for gaining entrance to medical school. This caused considerable anxiety for Bill's father, who worried he would 'flop out' in his final exams and never become a doctor.

After Founder's Day in June each year, Bill's parents took him for a meal at Veeraswamy, in Piccadilly, the oldest Indian restaurant in London. The first-floor dining rooms overlook the graceful architecture of Regent Street, but for Bill it was the 'swish décor and chaps wandering around in colourful turbans' that were the most memorable aspects of this restaurant. 'Usually it was just the three of us, but sometimes Kathy joined us,' says Bill of the younger of his two sisters. Kathy was now working in the music department of Harrods department store in Knightsbridge and would soon be leaving for a trip abroad with a girlfriend.

Bill's older sister Eleanor was engaged to a young doctor named Richard Marshall, who she met on a physiotherapy placement at St Bartholomew's, or Barts, as this hospital is often called. Bill and Bob were to be ushers at their wedding in the spring of 1960 at St Gregory's in Dawlish, with a reception in a marquee at Whickham Lodge afterwards.

John had shown Eleanor and Kathy 'just the rudiments' of driving while he was conducting his home visits and now he did the same for Bill and Bob. One of the twins' more memorable driving lessons was to the Dawlish cemetery at dusk because their father was required to attend the post-mortem of one his patients in the morgue. All it needed were some carrion crows circling and cawing to complete the eerie scene for the boys, who were told to wait in the car. 'After three quarters of an hour we saw dad emerge from the morgue. Then he broke into a trot and started running towards the headlights of the car,' says Bill, who later discovered that his father disliked these after-dark visits to the cemetery as much as he and Bob did.

Although he did not consider himself a 'brilliant letter writer', Bill did write home about four or five times a term. Bob was a boarder at the Kings College, Taunton, in Somerset. Jane always used to smile when she received a letter from one of her sons as she knew there would soon be a letter from her other son with very similar news. She put this down to a certain amount of mental telepathy between them. 'When we were at school we did the same sort of thing,' says Bill. 'I threw the javelin for Carr House at the athletic carnival and was a member of the Second VI team for tennis. Then I would find out that Bob had done javelin and tennis as well.'

Bill earned successes on the tennis courts and the athletics fields, but it was difficult for him to match the stellar sporting success of his father, who had been awarded the MacFarlane Cup for best all-round athlete in his final year at Epsom College.[4] A highlight of Bill's sporting career was playing in the Carr House rugby team in 1959, when they beat Propert in the House Cup final one Wednesday after school. Bill played several seasons of rugby for the Epsom Third XV, but narrowly missed out on selection for a prized position on the College First XV team. While he found this decision highly annoying, surely it couldn't affect his chances of attending one of the top London medical schools?

* * *

In his final year at Epsom College, Bill became a prefect. While the other boys in the house only had a toyce, he was given a 'bin' – half a room divided by a curtain with a desk and couch. Fagging was still in practice and Bill could have got his own back, but he was nice to the junior boy who looked after him. Other privileges included prefects' suppers and the prefects' dance, for which partners were sent across from Rosebery School, a well-known girls' school in the district. Bill hums the tunes as he remembers dancing the 'Duke of Wellington' and the 'Gay Gordons', but a disappointing aspect of the evening was only being paired up with one girl.

Bill and one of his fellow Carr House prefects, Bush, became involved with the debating society which met in the Barnes Wallis Library. The society normally had an attendance of about ten people, but the numbers swelled considerably when Bill became the president and chose as the topic for a debate: Was Hitler famous or infamous? 'It was just so outrageous,' says Bill, grinning broadly as he recalls the capacity crowd of 150 people. Bush asserted for the affirmative, 'We may think that Hitler is nasty now but he may end up like Napoleon … the French people like him now.' Bill recalls that the masters went 'ballistic' when the motion that Hitler was famous was nearly carried. They gave Bill and his teammates a stern lecture about the kind of statement they were making.

The shy first former who was picked on when he first arrived at the college was now a confident senior. Bill thinks that his separation from Bob may have been for the best. 'Perhaps it was the making of me … the making of both of us. If Bob and I had both attended Epsom College and tried to defend our patch, things may have worked out quite differently.' The principal of Epsom College, Henry Franklin, who Bill found to be a 'very daunting, distant and elderly character', had been against the idea of the Gibson twins attending the college together from the start.

The last five or so weeks of the school year were a busy time for the students, because they had to prepare for their exams while the cricket season was well underway. Bill replaced his grey flannels with cricket whites and played quite a lot of cricket during his last summer at Epsom College. 'I was given some acknowledgment for my wicket keeping but it was too late,' says Bill, whose name never appeared in gold letters on the board displaying the students awarded with 'Colours', because he wasn't selected for the Firsts team in either cricket or rugby.

Bill and his brother both thought their father placed even more emphasis on sport than he did on their schoolwork. Perhaps this was because John Gibson knew from personal experience that sporting success at school was an expectation of some of the more traditional hospital medical schools in London, such as St Mary's and St Thomas's. John's 'Colours' had helped earn him a sporting scholarship to St Thomas's but he had no influence at this hospital now.

There were also several doctors on the maternal side of Bill's family, including one of Ammy's brothers, William Kellock, who had been a prominent surgeon at the Middlesex Hospital in London. It was just as well that Professor Brian Windeyer, the dean of the

Middlesex Hospital Medical School, offered Bill a place because he hadn't applied anywhere else. When the results of the A-levels were released, Bill was awarded the Asher Asher Prize for biology and a full scholarship – the Freer Lucas Scholarship – to the Middlesex Hospital. This represented a saving for Bill's parents of £60 per year in tuition fees for the duration of his degree. 'Dad was pleased that I did well academically and he forgave me my lack of sporting prowess.'

* * *

This would be the last completely carefree summer holiday that Bill spent with Bob. One of the noticeable differences in appearance between the brothers – who both now stood around five feet nine inches (175 centimetres) in height – was that Bill had his blond hair parted on one side and Bob had it parted on the other. Like mirror images of each other, they also held their beer mugs in opposite hands. Bill and Bob sometimes pretended to be each other for their summer jobs, such as selling ice-creams and putting out deck-chairs at the holiday parks of Dawlish Warren, but playing the imitation game while driving a van led to some trouble with the police.

Bill was employed to drive a delivery van for a friend of his father's, Seymour Laxson, who had a business selling smallgoods and was reputedly 'a wheeler and dealer'. One day when Bob asked Bill if he could drive Mr Laxson's van, a policeman spotted him driving down a one-way street in the wrong direction. He waved him over and said, 'Son, do you have your driver's licence?' Bob didn't have it so he signed Bill's name on a piece of paper and promised to report to the police station the next day. Bill spent hours that evening practising Bob's style of signature and says, 'The policeman let me off, but he was very suspicious'.

The twins were desperate to have their own set of wheels so they were very pleased when their father's practice partner, Bob Sammons, gave them a 1932 MG J2 sports car which had belonged to his son Anthony and was now in pieces. Bill restored the car's electrics and remembers acting as the assistant to Bob, who fortunately was 'good with engines'. Bob would keep tinkering away on their car during his school holidays but Bill had to give up on the project. He was about to go up to London and start his medical degree in one of the most exciting decades imaginable for a young person: the 1960s.

Bill's separation from Bob during their senior years of schooling made it easier for them to go their separate ways at the end of this holiday, although Bill considers that breaking their total dependence on each other had come at a price. 'When we started at Beacon School we were twins, but by the time we finished boarding school we were more like brothers.'

CHAPTER 3

A medical qualification

There was a circuit of engagement
parties around that time, as most
of us were nearly ready to qualify.

Bill Gibson

Throughout the history of the British Isles, more than eighty hospitals have existed in London.[1] Bill Gibson worried that he perhaps was 'the kiss of death' to the ten or so hospitals where he trained because most of them have since been redeveloped or reduced to piles of rubble. Among the hospitals doomed for demolition was the Middlesex, where Bill completed his medical degree. Bill describes the H-shaped building fronting Mortimer Street, located in the trendy Soho district, as both 'very lovely and very Georgian' but appearances can be deceptive. The hospital was actually a replica of the original 1757 building, and had been completed in 1935.[2]

The induction tour for the sixty freshers in Bill's year concluded towards the rear of the hospital's 3-acre site at the brand new Middlesex Hospital Medical School in Cleveland Street. It was a grey October morning in 1962 when Bill pushed for the first time through the swing doors of this square-set, glass-gleaming building to hear the opening address by the Dean, Sir Brian Windeyer. There would be no settling-in time for Bill. As a result of his A-levels in biology, physics and chemistry, he was placed in the second stage (2nd MB) of his medical degree, allowing him to skip at least the first twelve months.

'We started dissecting human corpses pretty well straight away,' recalls Bill, who enjoyed the demonstrations by his tall, thin Anatomy Professor, Sir Eldred Walls. 'There were four of us to each body and you had to dissect away the skin and muscles, then the arm, shoulder and hand.' Over the course of eighteen months, each group dissected a whole body, which Bill observed 'had been preserved in formalin so long it was like cutting into plasticine'.

During physiology lectures, in a large raked auditorium on the ground floor of the medical school, Bill remembers that Professor Eric Neil would ask the students questions to see if they were paying attention. 'There was this chap in our year named Green and one day Professor Neil looked directly at him and shouted, "Green, PBI!" to which Green replied, "No, sir, my initials are PBW", or something like that. He was supposed to say "protein bound iodine", which is a thyroid test, and everyone in the lecture theatre thought this was tremendously funny.' During another lecture, Professor Neil told the students about an island where there was a ratio of eight men for every woman. 'There were only half a dozen girls in our year. One of them was terribly offended by this story and started walking towards the door,' says Bill, who breaks into a grin as he adds that Professor Neil then called after her, 'There's no point rushing to go there now. They will all still be there in a couple of days' time.'

In the evenings Bill caught the Tube from Oxford Circus to Wembley Park and descended the same steps as fans attending football matches at the Wembley Stadium, which he remembers dominating the dusk skyline with its flag-topped twin towers. It was a walk of nearly a mile from the Tube to the 'typical semi-detached' of his landlady, Mrs Jones, who for 30 shillings a week made his bed, his breakfast and his supper.

One evening Mrs Jones gave Bill a message that his father had suffered a heart attack but by the time he returned his mother's call, 'the crisis was over'. Jane told him that his father, who was only fifty-one, was having a couple of weeks' forced bed rest at the Royal Devon & Exeter Hospital. 'They didn't have stents and bypasses then so he was restricted in what he could do,' says Bill, who adds that his father had previously been 'a county squash player for Devon'.

On Sundays Bill liked to do 'something sedate' such as frequenting the coffee shops in the northern London suburb of Hampstead with Andrew Alison, a friend from Epsom College. But on Saturdays he liked to be near all the action of Soho. Bill associates London in the 1960s with the Carnaby Street fashion precinct. This was the place to be seen and buy his favourite bell-bottom trousers in the boutiques of designers such as John Stephen. Just around the corner in Oxford Street there was the Marquee Club, where Bill sometimes went with friends from the hospital to listen to bands at night.

There were several medical students with whom Bill became friends at the Middlesex, including Bernie Ribeiro, whose father was the Ambassador for Ghana to the USA. As members of the Middlesex Hospital Rugby Club, they enjoyed playing against other hospitals in the greater London area. After one of their rugby training sessions, Bill and Bernie were told to shower and be 'dressed presentably' because the Queen Mother was visiting the hospital. They rushed into the changing room but there wasn't time for a shower so they pulled on their crumpled clothes and stood at the back of the group, where they hoped not to be noticed. 'It was all right for Bernie with his dark skin,' says Bill with a wide grin, 'but with me the mud was pretty obvious.'

The Queen Mother, followed by an entourage of about eight people, parted the crowd and walked straight towards the filthy pair to say hello and shake Bernie's hand. The *Guardian* described the Queen Mother as having 'the knack of giving the most pretentious function the air of a jumble sale'[3] and Bill found her to be just as delightfully informal the day he met her. 'She was charming, she was lovely, she didn't turn a hair; it was the powers that be at the hospital. You could see the vice-chancellor of the University and Professor Eldred Walls bristling up because we were contrary to instructions.'

A few times a year, Bill caught the Tube to Twickenham, the home of English rugby union. Bill attended matches with his father, who had caught the train up from Dawlish with friends such as Roger Blackney, Dougy Knight and Seymour Laxson. 'Each time the English team scored, their supporters broke into the chorus of "Land of Hope and Glory",' says Bill, who uses a deep voice to demonstrate how they sang this patriotic song.

During Bill's first summer holidays he went home to Dawlish for the wedding of his sister Kathy to Martin Lundmark, a school headmaster from Calgary in Alberta, Canada. As they had after Eleanor's wedding, Kathy's parents hosted her reception in a marquee in the garden of Whickham Lodge. After the newlyweds returned to Canada, Bill and Bob borrowed their mother's Mini Minor and went on their first camping trip to the French Riviera. At the camping ground they were told to come back the next day, so they went down to the beach, where they had a few drinks with some young French men and their girlfriends. When Bill and Bob woke around 11 am, their sleeping bags were surrounded by a ring of sand, and beyond that a beach crowded with sunbakers.

After returning from this adventure, Bob went abroad and backpacked his way around Europe. 'Bob was very good at going off with a backpack and £20 in his pocket and having a wonderful time,' says Bill, who regrets not 'going off for a while' himself before starting medical school.

* * *

Bill found living with Mrs Jones 'a bit restrictive', so at the end of his first year of medical school he moved into a terrace house in Gilden Crescent, Kentish Town, owned by the father of another medical student, James Bramble. 'Jimmy had the best bedroom in the house, next to the kitchen, whereas I was on the top floor of this old house that was three or four storeys high but only this wide,' says Bill, holding his hands a few feet apart. Bill shared his top-floor room with John Gartside, an older medical student from his year, who became a good friend and introduced him to gambling. Bill also socialised with a housemate his own age, Patrick Thomas, who had an IQ of more than 150 and was brilliant at both bridge and poker. During card games in the common room of the medical school, the students played for money, which Bill says 'was always a bad idea with Pat because he could remember the order of every card in the pack'.

With all the excitement of living in London, Bill found it difficult to 'get down to study', so for the ten weeks leading up to his 2nd MB exam he had to study in the library every night from 6 pm until 10 pm. The reward for passing this 'very scary' exam was being allowed to see patients on the wards for the next three years. While he rotated through about a dozen medical specialties, Bill wore a little white coat which ended at his waist and he referred to as a 'bum freezer'.

Bill was placed in the same 'firm' of six to ten medical students as John Graham, who had completed the theory component of his degree at Oxford University. During their psychiatry term, Bill and John were permitted to sit in on psychotherapy sessions conducted by Professor Heinz Wolff. John Graham can still remember his friend's wise words about this specialty: 'As far as Bill could work out, psychiatry was about people not getting enough of something or else getting too much. I thought that was perfectly reasonable at the time and I still do.'

At six months in duration, one of the longest clinical terms Bill and John completed was general surgery. The two of them felt proud when they survived their first autopsy without vomiting, although Bill remembers feeling 'woozy' during his first amputation. 'I had to hold onto a man's leg while the consultant sawed it off and then I had to carry it to the other side of the theatre,' says Bill. He didn't faint on that occasion but he did another day in the lift after donating blood. 'I wasn't as bad as Doc Martin', says Bill, referring to the blood-averse doctor in the BBC television comedy series of the same name. 'At least, I got used to the sight of other people's blood; it was my own that was the problem.'

The medical students also carried out minor duties such as collecting blood in the wards and the outpatient clinics, which were conducted in a former workhouse only a few doors from the medical school in Cleveland Street. Fronted by a distinctive brick wall, with sweeping curves between each pillar, this utilitarian building is believed to be the template for the workhouse in Charles Dickens's *Oliver Twist*.[4] It was now a busy Outpatients Department not far from the throng of shoppers on Oxford Street.

One of the clinics Bill attended in this Outpatients Department was Ear, Nose and Throat (ENT). Bill explains that the full name of this specialty is actually otorhinolaryngology, from the Greek for ear (*otos*), nose (*rhinos*) and throat (*laryngos*). The ENT consultants allowed the medical students to peer into the ear canal with an auriscope (also known as an otoscope) which had inbuilt illumination and magnification. William Lund showed the students a series of slides about some delicate new surgical procedures involving the middle ear which had been made possible by the operating microscope. No particular specialty had leapt out at Bill until this ENT term, and he wondered if perhaps he had found his calling.

Bill was also instructed in the use of another instrument, an ophthalmoscope, to check the back of the eye for thromboses (tiny clots) on the retina, which he says are 'a sign of death'. One day, when someone had died on the ward, Bill pulled aside the curtain and snuck inside to see if the instrument worked. 'I had my hand on the man's chest and just as I was peering into his eye, the corpse let out an "argh" sound which was probably the last bit of air being expelled from his lungs.' Bill didn't stop running until he reached the common room of the medical school. It brought back memories of the evening he and his brother had sat in a car in the Dawlish cemetery waiting for their father to emerge from the morgue.

Bill was excited when Bob told him he was moving to London and would be bringing with him their MG J2. Bill says that 'finished' was not a good descriptor for this sports car, which still 'leaked oil as well as having bald tires and defective brakes'. After sharing a bedroom with Bill and also John Gartside at Gilden Crescent for about four months, Bob decided that he wanted to be nearer to his course at the College of Estate Management, so he moved to Paddington.

The social scene in arty Paddington was much better than shabby old Kentish Town. Bob soon had a girlfriend named Anne who worked for the actress Jane Asher, and also the Beatles, 'in some capacity'. When Bob told Bill that he had been to the Abbey Road studios and met the Beatles, including Jane's boyfriend Paul McCartney, it didn't seem very significant. 'Thinking about it now, it was *immensely* important,' says Bill, who had a fleeting encounter with the band himself about a block away from the Middlesex

Hospital. Bill was walking up Charlotte Street, just off the Tottenham Court Road, when he noticed four mod-looking guys in Carnaby-style clothing running in and out of the disused Scala Theatre. The Beatles had become an overnight sensation a few years before with their hit single 'Love Me Do' and were filming their black-and-white biopic *A Hard Day's Night*. Bill chuckles as he recalls an old fellow in the crowd saying that the band was rubbish and their tunes would never last. Bill comments, 'You can always get something wrong, I suppose'.

There was a thriving folk music scene in a heritage-listed pub directly across the road from the medical school, the King and Queen, which has been the 'exam results waiting room' for doctors in training for hundreds of years.[5] A young Bob Dylan performed his first London gig at this pub, on the corner of Cleveland and Foley Streets, and the Gibson brothers chose it as the venue for drinks to celebrate their twenty-first birthdays, with friends from both their sets.

When Ammy died in 1962, she left Bill and Bob £2000 each in her will. Now, three years later, their inheritance could be released with capital growth. The big-ticket item purchased by Bill was a black MG MGB sports car, whereas Bob bought a bright yellow Lotus Elan, which he boasted could go from nought to 100 miles per hour between two sets of traffic lights in Bayswater, near his flat in Paddington.

On their next trip home to Dawlish, Bill and Bob received gold signet rings from their father, who said they were part of their Irish family heritage. On the flat surface of the rings is an engraving of a pelican, which Bill says 'in mythology is said to feed the flesh and blood from its own chest to its starving young'. Bill knew that his family had some connection to Edward Gibson, who was raised to the peerage as Baron Ashbourne by Queen Victoria in 1885 for 'the good deeds he did for the Irish', including drafting the *Ashbourne*

Act, which allowed tenants to purchase their land. However, Bill thinks his father was 'fantasising' when he told him that the Ashbourne title might come down their line if the current heir, a Royal Navy commander in his thirties, never married. 'It all became immaterial a few years later when I read in the *Times* that the Honourable Edward Gibson was married and now had sons. I never thought about the title again after that.'

* * *

Medical revues are an institution in the United Kingdom but Bill had never felt sufficiently talented at singing or acting to involve himself with any of the concerts or musicals mounted in the medical school's auditorium. Then one night at the King and Queen, someone asked Bill if he would take part in the next dramatic production. 'The fellow must have picked just the right moment to ask me because for some strange reason I said yes. It turned out to be one of the best decisions I ever made.'

In the spring of 1966 Bill appeared in the Middlesex Hospital's production of Robert Bolt's play *A Man for All Seasons*. Bill played the part of the assistant to the Spanish Ambassador, who, he says, 'only had about three lines of dialogue and wasn't one of the main characters by a long chalk. I was blond at the time, so Alex dyed my hair black and made me up to look Spanish.'

Alexandra Carr worked as a medical secretary in the Nuclear Medicine department of the hospital and it is very unlikely that Bill would have met her if he had not taken part in the play. He found a book listing restaurants that offered a meal for two people for less than £1. It didn't take many of these dinners for Bill and Alex to discover how much they had in common, including the fact that they were both twenty-one and both war-time babies. 'Alex is thirteen days older than me,' says Bill, beaming as he recalls the early days of their courtship. 'Our fathers both served in World War II, so we may have even been conceived on the same day if they were both granted the same leave, nine months before D–Day.'

On his first visit to Alex's parents in a northern suburb of London, Bill discovered that Peter Carr served as a photographer for the Royal Air Force during the war and took photographs from the air of destroyed cities. Elvira Carr told Bill about how she used ration cards to buy tins of IXL peaches from Australia as a treat for Alex and her older brother, Edward. Bill comments, 'These were the kind of luxuries that were difficult to find during the war'.

One weekend Bill took Alex down to Devon to meet his parents, who he says 'definitely approved'. John thought that Alex would be very good for Bill, just as Jane had always been wonderfully supportive of him. Being absent-minded was evidently a family trait shared by Bill, Bob and their father John, so they all needed strong, organised women to take care of them.

Bill also took Alex to meet Con, who was living with her daughter Joan and son-in-law Victor Ralston in the southern London suburb of New Maldon. Con thought Bill and Alex were already engaged and kept alluding to this, which was perhaps wishful thinking on her part. Bill's next visit to New Maldon was to attend Con's funeral and cremation, which he found 'quite gruesome when the coffin descended towards the fire'. It was not the way Bill wanted to remember his grandmother, who had lived her life with such panache right up to the end.

The consultant Bill was attached to for his orthopaedics term, Rodney Sweetnam, also had a certain style about him. This included his habit of wearing a red carnation in his jacket lapel. Sweetnam would later be knighted when he became the orthopaedic surgeon to Queen Elizabeth II but Bill knew him when he was in his late thirties.[6] Sweetnam only said a few words to each of the sixty or so patients in his Orthopaedics Clinic, which he conducted so briskly

that Bill recalls it just went, 'boom, boom, boom'. Bill liked the way
it was possible to fix the bones and make them straight with the help
of weights and pulleys, and wavered on whether he should choose
orthopaedics instead of ENT as his specialty.

Eye-catching dress was a characteristic common to *all*
consultants, not just Rodney Sweetnam. Rather than wearing a
white coat, as was the norm for the other medical staff, Bill says the
consultants paraded around like peacocks in their three-piece suits
with 'little handkerchiefs poking out of their top pockets'.

At the end of each year, the medical students chose some of the
hospital consultants to send up in the 'Manic Depressives Christmas
Concert', which was held in the auditorium at the medical school.
Bill recalls that humorous lyrics about the consultants would be set
to the tunes of songs such as 'I Am the Very Model of a Modern
Major-General' from *Pirates of Penzance*. He would not normally
have been involved but Alex was singing in the chorus of *Beyond the
Syringe*, which was a play on the name of the long-running West
End revue *Beyond the Fringe*. Bill's contribution to the Christmas
concert was running the bar with a medical student from his year
named Hilmar Warenius, who played in the band.

Bill's fellow medical student and flatmate Patrick Thomas had
recently asked him to be his best man. Bill had quite a few other
friends from the Middlesex Hospital who were also making plans to
marry. 'There was a circuit of engagement parties around that time,
as most of us were nearly ready to qualify.'

About once or twice a month Bill and Alex went out for a meal
with Bob. One evening, Bill was strangely insistent that the three of
them go to 'the hospital pub', as he called the King and Queen.
While Alex went to the powder room, Bill confided to his brother,
'I'm going to propose to Alex tonight'.

On 24 May 1967, two weeks after announcing his engagement
to Alex, Bill qualified from the University of London and was

presented with a certificate stating: 'Bachelor of Medicine and Bachelor of Surgery'. Achieving the letters 'MBBS' after his name had been 'an incredible amount of work' but Bill still needed at least twelve months of clinical training before he could be registered as a medical practitioner and practise independently.

It was prestigious to work in the hospital where you had trained but there were only sufficient positions at the Middlesex Hospital for about a quarter of the students in Bill's year. He felt very fortunate to be appointed as a houseman, reporting to the consultants in the Department of Otolaryngology. Bill thought this role was 'sending a message to the world' that he was interested in ENT.

Duties for a houseman included looking after patients on the wards and attending ENT clinics in the Outpatients Department in Cleveland Street, which was next door to the Ferens Institute of Otolaryngology. The Ferens was well-known for its clinical research, including the groundbreaking histological studies of the ear – in which thin slices of tissue were viewed under a microscope – performed by the otologist (ear specialist) Charles Hallpike in 1938. Hallpike demonstrated that patients with Menière's disease have an excess of fluid in a compartment of their inner ears.[7]

In the operating theatres, Bill was allowed to do simple tasks such as cutting the sutures for senior surgeons, including William Lund. The tonsillectomy was still a mainstay of the department and Bill also assisted Lund with a relatively new operation to restore the hearing of people with conductive hearing loss, which was the cause of Beethoven's deafness. If a tiny bone in the middle ear, called the stapes, becomes stiff and cannot vibrate in response to sound, surgeons were now able to replace it with a Teflon piston. Bill would later meet John Shea Jr, from Memphis, Tennessee, who was the first surgeon to successfully perform the stapedectomy operation. Afterwards he became a celebrity in the United States, appearing on the cover of *Life* magazine.[8]

Bill needed to be on call for after-hours work so he moved into Berners Hostel, directly opposite the Middlesex Hospital in Berners Street. To show that he was already qualified but not yet a registered doctor Bill replaced his white 'bum freezer' with a long white coat with a blue checked collar, which he says was 'not unlike the police checkerboard pattern'. He received free food and board and was paid nearly £500 for his six-month placement at the hospital.

Bill felt sufficiently wealthy to book tickets for himself and Alex, at £50 per person, for a ski trip to the pretty Austrian town of Alpbach with its traditional wooden chalets. For the *après ski*, Bill and Alex accompanied the eight or so other couples from the Middlesex Hospital to enjoy entertainment of the 'oom-pah-pah' variety, which Bill recalls was 'just a couple of guys singing in German, accompanied by an accordion and a lot of thigh slapping'.

A houseman who worked with Bill in the Department of Otolaryngology, Jonathan Hazell, would later reflect on these early days of their training when 'minds are wide open and you really can be fired up by enthusiastic teachers'.[9] Of the two ENT consultants Bill reported to, it was the head of the department, Sir Douglas Ranger, who took him 'under his wing' and encouraged him to become an ENT specialist. Bill thought he might be interested in laryngology (throat surgery) but that was before he assisted Ranger in an operation on a man whose throat had been ravaged by cancer. 'The operation isn't performed any more but they used to bring the stomach up through the chest and anastomose it [connect it surgically] to the back of the throat. As far as operations go, it was pretty mega.'

Bill noted that the patient was making slow progress after his surgery and was still having trouble swallowing a couple of weeks later. 'The poor chap threw himself out of the window, and fell eight stories before impaling himself on the spiked fence surrounding the hospital,' says Bill. 'After the body was removed, the fire brigade had to be brought in to hose off the remaining blood and gore, because it was a major thoroughfare.'

* * *

Unlike his houseman position at the Middlesex, Bill's six-month placement at Bethnal Green Hospital was not intended to look good on his résumé; however, it provided him with a unique opportunity to treat the people of the East End. 'Nowhere in London was as poor as the East End,' says Bill, who arrived at Bethnal Green during the depths of winter. He recalls that patients were brought into casualty suffering from hypothermia, who were 'half frozen to death because they couldn't afford to buy coal or food'. Bill worked for a consultant with the reassuring name of Richard Balme but no tincture could help people in this state. Bill was advised to leave them in a room to warm up very slowly, and sometimes they lived. He recalls the 'very unfortunate case' of an old lady who was pronounced dead but then woke up in the morgue and had to be brought back up in the elevator from the basement to the ward.

There were wards in each of the eleven red brick pavilions of Bethnal Green Hospital, which had opened in 1900 as an infirmary for the inhabitants of workhouses and still had a very 'workhousy' feel when Bill arrived early in 1968. Some of the wards had verandahs to provide ventilation for patients with tuberculosis (TB), which was finally 'losing its grip' by the mid-1960s, due to antibiotics such as sulphonamides and streptomycin. One of Bill's TB patients was Reggie Kray, who, along with his twin brother Ronnie, had a fearsome reputation as the standover men of the East End. They would both later serve jail terms.

The arched brick entrance to Bethnal Green Hospital – all that remains today – faces Cambridge Heath Road. Running along the rear of the hospital was Russia Lane. As this name suggests, there was great cultural diversity in the East End including, as Bill recalls, 'a good mix of Russians, Dutch and Germans'. There was also a large Orthodox Jewish population and an emotional experience for Bill was treating survivors of the Nazi concentration camps. When survivors rolled up their sleeves so he could take their blood, Bill saw a horizontal line of identification numbers tattooed on their forearms. If they saw him staring at the line of numbers, they would tell him, 'I survived the Holocaust'.

The only details of the concentration camp Bill's father would reveal to him was the dreadful smell of death as he helped to liberate the survivors. Thinking back to his senior year at Epsom College, Bill hoped the Jewish people at his school were not too upset by his choice of debate topic. He doesn't think he realised at the time what the detainees of the camps had been through.

When Bill finished up at Bethnal Green he had completed his obligatory twelve months of post-qualification training. He was a registered doctor and theoretically could hang up his shingle straight away and become a general practitioner but he had decided to become a surgeon. However many years this would take, juggling a job with the study and exams required to become a Fellow of the Royal College of Surgeons, Bill would be doing it as a married man.

As a wedding gift for Alex, Bill had a replica made of his mother's ring – a blue sapphire engraved with the bird in the family crest, which he thinks looks more like a stork than a pelican. Bill smiles to himself as he recalls that his engagement to Alex lasted for exactly thirteen months and thirteen days. 'It wasn't planned that way ... we realised after the wedding. We're also thirteen days apart in age so it must be our lucky number.'

CHAPTER 4

Fellow of the College of Surgeons

The examiners brought their own patients with them to the viva, so you had to be very diplomatic and say things such as, 'Oh that's very nice surgery; beautifully done.'

Bill Gibson

A photo from Saturday 15 June 1968 shows the best man, Bob Gibson, pinning a carnation to Bill's lapel outside St Mary's Church of England at Harrow on the Hill. Standing shoulder to shoulder, dressed in matching dark grey morning suits, each brother resembles a reflection of the other. Having your marriage ceremony in a church more than 900 years old is romantic enough, but as Bill and Alex led their guests to the reception they passed a memorial to Lord Byron, who in his student days had sat under an elm tree in this churchyard to compose his poetry.

Later in the evening, as the wedding guests clustered around the second of Bill's cars, a blue Mini Van, he turned the key in the ignition. Nothing happened. 'Not that old chestnut,' Bill thought to himself. It didn't take long to work out that Alex's older brother had switched the leads around. 'Edward nearly blew the thing up,' says Bill, shaking his head. The weary couple eventually drove off towards a hotel near Heathrow airport in anticipation of their morning flight to Italy. Bill remembers that he and Alex had fallen asleep when the shrill ring of the telephone woke them with a start. 'It was Bob. I remember him ringing up about 11 o'clock at night to ask if anything had happened yet. We had gone through a wedding and to be woken by your brother asking impertinent questions – it was the height of rudeness,' says Bill, chuckling as he remembers the call that capped off a wonderful day.

After the newlyweds returned from their package holiday on the crowded beaches of the Mediterranean, they would be moving out of London to start their new lives and Bill's career as a registered medical practitioner. In preparation for their move to England's equivalent of the French Riviera, Bill packed the small amount of goods and chattels he and Alex owned into the back of his Mini Van. He included the physiology and anatomy textbooks that would constitute the 'light reading' for the first part of his surgery exams, known as the Primary Fellowship or simply 'the Primary'.

They would be starting married life in a small apartment with its own kitchenette at the back of Bill's parents' home in Dawlish, where Con had once stayed during her extended visits. There would be few opportunities for moonlit walks along the coastal path because Bill was expected to live in at the Royal Devon & Exeter (RD&E) Hospital, which was 12 miles from Dawlish. Bill had every third weekend off plus Wednesday afternoons, but he needed to be back in the residents' quarters by midnight. This didn't leave much time for Alex.

Bill's first position as a house surgeon fitted perfectly with his study plans. He learned a great deal in the operating theatres of a second Exeter hospital – the Exeter City Hospital – with the general surgeon, Henry 'Dendy' Moore. 'Dendy loved his vascular surgery and would spend hours stitching blood vessels together. If the blood wasn't getting through to the patient's legs, we would put in some grafts,' says Bill, explaining that atheromas are one of the main causes of blocked arteries. 'These fatty deposits can be present anywhere in your body, not just your heart.'

The RD&E Hospital was located in a two-storeyed Victorian building with open vistas of Exeter, which Bill considers to be a 'very historic' city despite having sustained extensive bomb damage during World War II. On the city outskirts, he saw evidence of Roman walls and paved roads, including the Wessex Way, which runs eastwards from Exeter towards London, past Stonehenge.

Alex liked coming into Exeter to see Bill during his breaks and enrolled in a lampshade-making class as a way of filling her spare time. When the instructor called the roll, there were two Mrs A Gibsons. Mrs Astrid Gibson, who is Norwegian, turned out to be married to the John Gibson who was head boy at Kings College, Taunton when Bob was a student in a more junior year at the same school. John Gibson was sporty, like Bill, and they enjoyed playing golf and squash together at the Exeter Golf and Country Club. The two couples also enjoyed socialising together in Exeter and have remained friends ever since.

Bill's parents rarely had the opportunity to go in to Exeter to see a movie and he was pleased to be able to do few locums so they could have a well-deserved night off from the medical practice. During one of these locums, Bill was called to the Great Western Railway Convalescent Home, located in Marine Parade, only a stone's throw from the Main Beach of Dawlish. On his arrival, he found the residents of the convalescent home, who had all been drivers or stokers on the railways, seated at tables of four, eating their evening meal. Bill noticed an old man lying on the floor next to an empty chair. 'A nurse was with the man using an ambubag to puff air into his lungs. She probably didn't want to do mouth to mouth, because he was as dead as a dodo,' says Bill. He was about to help the nurse move the corpse to a side room when one of the men from the same table motioned to the dead man's plate and asked, 'Is 'e dead yet, Doc?' When Bill replied in the affirmative, the man started to apportion the neglected dinner between the other three plates, and stated, 'Well, 'e won't be awanting his dinner, then.'

The Devon accent must be very easy to pick up, because Bill says that his father, who was brought up in Birmingham, ended up sounding quite Devonian. The same thing happened whenever Bill came home to Devon for more than a couple of weeks. If Alex made a comment about his accent, Bill would say, 'I'm not talk'n different, am I, m'dear?'

After his stint with Dendy Moore, Bill worked for an innovative orthopaedic surgeon, Freddy Durbin, in the department that was currently developing the Exeter prosthetic hip. For a second time Bill considered choosing orthopaedics as his surgical specialty. He also worked in Accident and Emergency (A&E), where 'everything seemed to happen at once.' He didn't even have a consultant to assist him, although Bill says that he was allowed to call for back-up from other departments.

> I treated the victims of motor vehicle accidents.
> There were lots of those, because cars were not as
> safe back then. We also saw retentions in the old
> men who came down to Devon by coach for their
> holidays. If the coaches got stuck on the Exeter by-
> pass, the poor old boys used to go into urinary
> retention and not be able to pee. They'd be brought

in to A&E *absolutely* desperate and we would put in
a catheter. They were so grateful; we could have
made a fortune out of those men.

Bill's sister Eleanor, her husband Richard Marshall and their daughters Sally, Catherine and Anna visited Dawlish during the summer holidays. They stayed in the front rooms of Whickham Lodge, while Bill and Alex stayed in their little flat at the back. During this visit, Richard suggested to Bill that he write up one of his interesting cases. The very first paper Bill published, entitled 'Avulsion of the upper limb', was about a man who had his arm ripped off in a mill.[1] 'Richard helped me to get it published in the *British Medical Journal*. It wasn't terribly novel, but it *was* a publication.'

On one of his evenings off, Bill and Alex drove with some other couples from the hospital over to a pub in the picture postcard village of Beer, on Devon's east coast. Bill recalls playing a game called skittles, which was very similar to ten pin bowling and involved rolling a wooden skittle down a 30-foot alley. Driving the 40-mile round trip to Beer on a Saturday evening for a game of skittles was nothing to Bill, who had once thrown two surfboards in the back of his MG sports car to drive with John Gibson the three hours each way to Cornwall 'just to go for a surf'.

Bill had dreams of staying longer in Devon, but there were several good reasons for returning to London. The first was that he wanted to sit the first part of his surgery exams at the Royal College of Surgeons (RCS). The second was that he and Alex were expecting their first child. Bill thought it would be nice for Alex to have her mother around during this special time, so they moved in with Peter and Elvira Carr.

* * *

There was plenty of room for them all at 8 Roxborough Avenue in Harrow on the Hill, even a garden with a little shed, where Peter Carr, who had already retired, could be heard tap, tapping away at his woodwork. Bill reluctantly replaced his MG MGB convertible with a Ford Cortina station wagon, because there wasn't enough room for the baby, let alone all the baby paraphernalia, in his sports car.

Although it was not close, Alex chose the very familiar Middlesex Hospital for her confinement in December 1969. Men were already allowed into the labour room at this time, but Bill recalls feeling anxious about Alex and the safe arrival of their firstborn, so at some point during the delivery he decided to wait outside. They named their first baby Laura Louise, who Bill says 'was very fair as a baby and still is today'.

By the time Bill held his baby girl in his arms for the first time, he was already a few months into his course at the RCS. From the Holborn tube station, it is only a short walk to the college, which occupies a handsome neoclassical sandstone building at one end of a large garden square called Lincoln's Inn Fields. Bill remembers the college having the feel of 'an old museum', with its floors and floors of wooden cabinets housing thousands of anatomical specimens comprising the Hunterian Museum. Although the museum's founder, John Hunter, is sometimes referred to as a 'barber surgeon', Bill considers him to be 'the father of surgery because he took it beyond the backstreets to become a profession'. Bill explains that the reason we still address a surgeon today as 'Mr' instead of 'Dr' is because in the 18th century, unqualified men would pay experts such as John Hunter to train them, and they received a diploma rather than a degree.

Fellows in training, like Bill, were allowed to wander around the Hunterian Museum whenever they liked. One of his favourite exhibits is the skeleton of the 7 foot 7 inch 'Irish giant' Charles Byrne, who died in 1783. In the same glass cabinet as Byrne's skeleton are his enormous boots and a sketch showing him towering above his fellow countrymen. Byrne's gigantism was the result of an overproduction of growth hormone by his pituitary gland and he was one of several giants who became quite famous because they exhibited themselves for show in England. Bill recalls there were rumours of 'skulduggery' regarding the way John Hunter acquired human remains, such as those of this giant, for which he was believed to have paid the large sum of £130 (more than £10000 today). 'The poor old Irish giant didn't want his skeleton displayed in a museum,' says Bill, 'he wanted to be buried in the Irish Sea. Hunter obviously bribed the undertaker with a lot more money.'

While Bill was studying at the RCS, he earned some money on Saturdays working at the North London Blood Transfusion Service, which took vans around the church halls in the area. 'We used to ask some simple questions, stick a cannula in and take a pint of blood,' says Bill, who didn't offer to donate himself. 'The others on the blood-collecting team thought it was funny that a doctor was squeamish about the sight of his own blood.' Since fleeing the labour room, Bill had realised that his squeamishness also extended to Alex and their children. One Saturday evening, Bill and Alex took baby Laura in 'a little carry cot' to the house of some friends for dinner. When they arrived home, the same friends telephoned to ask, 'Do you think you've forgotten something?'

When Bill first came up from Devon to Harrow on the Hill, he had attempted his Fellowship exam with only the knowledge he had gleaned from textbooks. After completing the 'Basic Surgical Sciences' course at the RCS, he had far more practical experience when he returned for a second time to the examination hall opposite the National Hospital for Nervous Diseases, where he was examined on every bone in the body 'from the head to the toe'.

Passing this Primary exam was Bill's passport to securing a more senior training position. After deciding that he definitely wanted to be an ENT surgeon, he was thrilled to become a senior house officer at what was widely considered to be the oldest ENT hospital in the world.[2] Founded in 1862 by Morell Mackenzie, a Scottish throat specialist, the branch of the Royal National Throat, Nose and Ear Hospital that was located at 32–33 Golden Square was usually referred to simply as 'Golden Square'. It was here, in this narrow, six-storey hospital in the heart of Soho that ENT emerged as a specialty in its own right, rather than being part of general surgery or linked to ophthalmology.

At the front of the Golden Square hospital there is a large traffic roundabout with a grassy area in the middle, measuring about 400 yards across. Bill recalls that people would sunbake and eat their sandwiches on the grass at lunchtime, but he thinks they might have chosen somewhere else to sit if they'd known that directly underneath them there was a 17th-century plague pit, 'into which the dead-carts had nightly shot corpses by scores'.[3] Between the roundabout and the hospital there was a car park with three 'very handy' car spaces reserved for the consultants.

Bill had a brief crossover with an eminent consultant named Sir Cecil Hogg, who was the aurist (ear specialist) to Queen Elizabeth II.[4] There was also a very elderly consultant, Mr Rotter, and a surgeon, Tony Bull, who Bill recalls did beautiful nose work. 'Rhinoplasty is a design thing, because you only take a little bit off here and there. I wasn't very interested in noses, or larynges either, for that matter,' says Bill, who had been put off throat surgery for life by Sir Douglas Ranger's horrific stomach pull-up operations.

As a relatively junior member of staff, Bill had to 'clerk' the patients, which involved booking them in and taking their clinical histories. He also watched and assisted with commonplace surgeries such as the removal of the tonsils, adenoids and polyps. The house surgeons took it turns to present departmental talks. One of the 'questions' Bill was asked to research was the treatment of facial palsies, which cause paralysis of the tissues and muscles innervated by the facial nerve.

When Bill was interviewed for a registrar's position at the Royal Free Hospital in 1971, he considered he only had 'an outside chance' because the other applicants were far more qualified. John Groves, who conducted the interview, asked Bill if he knew anything about facial palsies. 'Before long we got way trapped on the topic. This seemed to please Dr Groves and he offered me the registrar's job,' says Bill, whose appointment surprised many of his peers. This was just one of several milestones in Bill's fairly rapid career progression, which can be described as a combination of good luck *and* good management.

* * *

During Bill's time as a registrar at the Royal Free Hospital, John Groves proved to be everything a great mentor should be: kind, generous and encouraging. However, he could also be eccentric. 'John was lovely, he was fantastic and he was my boss most of the time, but we [the junior staff] referred to him as "Granny Groves" because he was very pedantic ... about everything, really. When he had a run-in with a theatre sister he didn't like, I used to sort of cower in the corner of the operating theatre.' Also contributing to his 'granny' status was Groves's habit of bringing his 'ancient old dog' with him to the hospital each day, where it sat in the back of his station wagon in the consultants' car park.

Bill also reported to a second John at the Royal Free, with the last name of Ballantyne. Anyone who works in the specialty of ENT would recognise 'Groves' and 'Ballantyne' as two of the three names in gold letters on the front cover of the weighty, multi-volume tome *Scott-Brown's Diseases of the Ear, Nose and Throat*, which the two Johns had assisted Walter Scott-Brown in editing from 1965 onwards.[5]

They would later ask Bill to contribute chapters to *Scott-Brown's,* which was one of the prescribed textbooks for the second part of his RCS Fellowship. While his Primary exam was very general and anatomical, the second part involved written examinations specifically related to ENT. He also had live interactions with one or more examiners, called 'vivas', for which his position at the Royal Free Hospital would provide the requisite practical experience.

Since Bill had started earning an income, he had been renting a flat for his family in Tufnell Park, near the Holloway Women's Prison. Now, after a year of saving for a deposit, Bill and Alex spotted a 'for sale' sign outside a brand new block of sixties-style flats called Fortier Court in Hornsey Lane. This flat was in walking distance of the Highgate shops and near a bridge over the Archway Road – a major thoroughfare for cars and coaches heading north out of London. Bill recalls their first mortgage being about £8000, which seemed to him like 'a massive amount of money to pay for such a boxy little place in a busy spot'. Their new abode was also near the Whittington Hospital, named after Richard 'Dick' Whittington, who served three terms as mayor of London in the 1300s. A statue of Dick's legendary cat, which Bill says supposedly told him to 'turn, turn, turn again' when he was about to head out of London, can be found in a protective wire cage on the side of the Archway Road.

Now that Bill had a mortgage to pay, he accepted an offer from one of the other registrars at the Royal Free Hospital to conduct his Friday evening surgery for him, treating the impoverished people of the East End. 'I worked for Archie Sherwood, as in Sherwood Forest. He paid me about five or ten pounds to turn up for a couple of hours to a general practice, run from a small house,' says Bill, who kept it going for a few years because it was easy money. Like Sherwood himself, many of his patients were Jewish and needed to be home by sunset to observe the Sabbath, so Bill used his moped to deliver medicines to the letterboxes of these families on his way home.

The Royal Free came into existence because of a young girl found 'dying of disease and hunger' on the steps of a Holborn church by the surgeon William Marsden in 1828.[6] The girl, who had been refused admission to three London hospitals, died in Marsden's arms and he determined to establish a hospital that treated the kind of patients others turned away. In Victorian times it was not only prostitutes and unmarried mothers who could not gain entry to hospitals, but also the 'truly destitute', since they were viewed as having 'moral failings'.[7] By the time Bill worked at the Royal Free, it was widely considered to be the most innovative of the twelve London teaching hospitals.

It was while working with John Groves at the Royal Free that Bill says he 'drifted into ears' as his particular area of interest in ENT. He became fascinated by the delicate microsurgery of the middle and inner ear made possible by the operating microscope, introduced a decade earlier by the Zeiss Optical Company. Bill was justifiably proud that ear surgeons were the first group to use a microscope to see minute structures clearly during surgery. The stapedectomy operation would not have been possible without magnification and Bill would later report in a clinical paper about the operating microscope that this operation achieved a success rate of over 90 per cent in restoring hearing.[8]

John Groves demonstrated to Bill another relatively new operation that required a microscope, called a 'tympanoplasty'. Bill would later meet the German surgeon who devised this operation.

> Horst Wüllstein was the first person to successfully graft a perforated eardrum. At first he used small patches of skin to repair the eardrums, but the skin used to give way, so then Wüllstein used the fascia covering a bundle of muscle fibres. Before these early grafts, there wasn't much that could be done for people with perforated ears.

As a registrar, Bill was allowed to perform minor operations on his own. He took the patient through the whole journey, from pre-operative checks, including their heart, to ensuring they had recovered sufficiently to be discharged from hospital. John Groves encouraged Bill to come up with his own ideas, even if they were only refinements to the established ENT methods. In one paper, Bill described a plastic speculum he placed into the ear canal prior to imaging studies to make it easier to identify anatomical structures such as the tiny stapes bone.[9] Bill describes this paper and another he wrote about an illuminated instrument which could be inserted into the throat[10] as 'helpful' but still not 'particularly novel'. Like every young medical researcher, he dreamed of discovering something that would make a difference to the clinical management of his patients.

Sometimes after finishing work for the day, Bill would have a drink with Bob at a pub near where he lived in Paddington, called the Warwick Castle. Bob surprised Bill one evening by bringing along a new girlfriend who was from Australia. 'There was a lady dressed all in black. Everything was black, even her hair,' says Bill. 'It was Jan. By the time I met her, she and Bob were already a firm item. The next thing we knew Bob was engaged and then he went to live in Australia.' For Bill, Bob's departure would feel like their separation when he went on his own to board at Epsom College all over again.

In anticipation of the birth of their second child in September 1971, Bill and Alex purchased a fully attached house in Claremont Road, Highgate for £17 000. The delivery room registrar for Alex's second confinement was someone from the year below Bill at the Middlesex Hospital, who he knew well enough to say 'hello' to in the corridor. When Bill told him that he and Alex were going to call their infant son Hugh, the registrar said, 'Oh that's nice. You named him after me.' Bill says that wasn't the case at all. 'So far there had been all girls in the family, because my sisters both have three daughters. We thought we'd call him Hugh Rea, as in "hoo-ray" for a boy. But we dropped the Rea,' says Bill. 'We spared him that and called him Hugh William instead.'

The same month Hugh was born, Bill sat the second part of his surgery Fellowship exam. He remembers colleagues who had already sat the viva warning him not to make any disparaging remarks about the patient's past surgical procedures. 'The examiners brought their own patients with them to the viva, so you had to be very diplomatic and say things such as, "Oh that's very nice surgery; beautifully done."'

Receiving the results of the Fellowship exam was a big moment after all these years of study so Bill took Alex with him to wait in the RCS library. As their gazes lifted from the book-lined walls to the panelled ceiling, with portraits of former surgeons hanging just underneath, they listened intently for Bill's number to be called. Bill had forgotten the number he'd written at the top of his exam papers and was worried he had missed out, but fortunately Alex remembered it and they soon realised with great excitement that he had passed.

* * *

Unlike Laura, who had been christened at St Mary's Church of England in Harrow on the Hill, for Hugh's christening Bill and Alex chose a church in Powderham, near Powderham Castle in Devon. Bill can't remember why they selected this chapel but he thinks perhaps his father's former colleague Douglas Peterkin must have known the vicar.

Bill loved bringing his family down to Dawlish for holidays by the sea where the children could make their sandcastles near the breakwater and his mother baked them treats such as his favourite treacle tart. Bill recalls that his father would tell him about the

Dawlish folk who had either retired or died. 'I preferred to hear about the engagement parties rather than the funerals,' says Bill, who nonetheless was generous about taking time to visit his father's retired medical colleagues, Douglas Peterkin and Bob Sammons.

His father and the other Dawlish doctors had been the role models for Bill while he was growing up. Now it was John Groves who was providing the inspiration and Bill always made sure to acknowledge him in any papers by using the pronoun 'we' when he reported their findings. He also acknowledged the staff of the other hospitals where he worked as part of his duties as a registrar at the Royal Free Hospital. These included the 'rather spooky' Badham Clinic, which was run from a former World War II morgue in Camden Town, and Hampstead General Hospital. In a couple of years' time, the Royal Free would move up to Hampstead as part of a drive to move some of the teaching hospitals out of the bustling centre of London. Bill should not have worried that he was the 'kiss of death' to the teaching hospitals in central London; there were simply too many.

Despite finding his boss pernickety at times, Bill describes the two years he spent with John Groves at the Royal Free as 'happy days'. Towards the end of this period, he was permitted to do his own research including a study of patients with facial palsy to determine the significance of someone's sense of taste to their prognosis. He presented his findings at the Royal Society of Medicine at No. 1 Wimpole Street in London's West End.

Like the RCS, the Royal Society of Medicine has beautiful libraries and museum-like exhibits such as the display of old-fashioned ENT instruments in the Toynbee Mackenzie Room. In addition to Morell Mackenzie, this room is named after another father of the ENT profession: Joseph Toynbee, who collected and studied thousands of temporal bones – the bones on either side of the skull which enclose the inner and middle ears. The society also hosts educational events for many branches, or 'sections' as they are called, of medicine. Bill spoke in the Otology Section, which, as he recalls, was conducted in a large hall with lots of 'fuddy duddys sitting in the front row who were about sixty years plus'. Many wore hearing aids and if they weren't enjoying the presentation they would pull them out and Bill could hear 'a buzzing sound'.

The talk Bill gave on facial palsies was the first of many he would deliver at the Royal Society of Medicine. It was very well received and afterwards John Groves introduced him to his friend Ellis Douek, an ENT consultant at Guy's Hospital. Douek asked Bill what he planned to do when he concluded his employment as a registrar at the Royal Free. He said he would put Bill's name forward to work with him at Guy's Hospital so he could do some original research towards a Doctorate of Medicine (MD).

'It was John Groves who first came up with the idea of me doing an MD,' says Bill. 'John said, "Everything is going a bit too fast. Why don't you go off and do something else for a year?"' John Groves had a point. Not only was Bill a fully qualified and registered medical practitioner by the age of twenty-three, but he had passed his surgery exams and been made a Fellow of the College of Surgeons by twenty-seven.

For his MD project, Groves suggested to Bill that he look into electrocochleography, a new method of testing the responses of the inner ear to external sounds. He also suggested that Bill go to Bordeaux, where this specialised form of electrophysiological testing was first developed. Bill hoped the eight weeks he spent living with his family in a small French resort town near Bordeaux would be a shorter version of the gap year he had missed out on before starting his medical degree.

CHAPTER 5

Taking a new direction

The doctorate of medicine was an optional extra that seemed like a good idea at the time. Not many people had this additional degree, so it potentially allowed me to stand out from the crowd.

Bill Gibson

In the summer of 1972, the Gibson family rented a white Spanish Mission-style villa in a town on the south-west coast of France, Arcachon, which Bill remembers as being 'quite small and touristic'. Each weekday Bill travelled the 40 kilometres from Arcachon to his electrophysiology course in the centre of Bordeaux using the car he had brought with him from London. 'I drove in my Renault 4, with its funny little gearstick sticking out of the dashboard, smoking Gitanes because these are the things you do in France!'

The Institut Georges Portmann is located at 114 Avenue d'Arès in a very medical quarter of Bordeaux, only a few blocks back from the Garonne River. Three generations of the Portmann family had taken it in turns to run this institute and Bill met both the current director Michel and his father Georges, who was in his eighties. Bill considers that it was Professor Georges Portmann who cemented the institute's reputation with his 'masterly surgical skills and pioneering studies on Menière's disease'.

Of all the conditions that can affect someone's ears and hearing, Menière's is perhaps the most debilitating. Bill would devote the rest of his career to learning more about this disease, named for the Frenchman Prosper Menière, who in 1861 described the following classic set of symptoms: sudden and recurring attacks of vertigo associated with nausea and vomiting, hearing loss, tinnitus and a blocked-up feeling in the affected ear.[1]

To simulate this disease in an animal species, Georges Portmann conducted experiments on sharks housed in large tanks at the University of Bordeaux's marine laboratories in Arcachon. Bill explains that Portmann chose sharks because they have an opening on the surface of their heads where it was possible for him to block off the lateral line. This blockage resulted in a surplus of fluid accumulating in the inner ears of the sharks and caused them to swim around in circles in a disoriented way. Georges Portmann employed a cinematographer to film lemon sharks displaying this bizarre behaviour, which is not unlike the unsteadiness experienced by patients with Menière's disease.

He performed the first operation on a Menière's sufferer in 1926, draining the excess fluid from the endolymphatic sac in the inner ear of a male telephone technician, with only the surgical equivalent of a gouge and hammer at his disposal.[2] Afterwards, the man's attacks of vertigo abated and he was once again able to climb the high poles to string telephone wires, which his trade required.

When Georges Portmann retired in 1967, his son Michel took over as director of the institute. The same year, Michel began offering ENT courses for English speakers which became known around the world as 'the otorhinolaryngology school in Bordeaux'. The course included demonstrations of temporal bone dissections and microsurgery techniques; however, Bill was primarily interested in the newer and more technologically challenging electrocochleography (ECochG), for which an electrical engineer was required to design and operate the equipment.

Bill met the engineer, Jean-Marie Aran, who in 1967 had co-authored with Michel Portmann the first article in this emerging field, which was published in the medical journal associated with the institute, *Revue de Laryngologie*.[3] Bill attended the course at the institute only five years after the publication of this seminal paper and would become one of the early adopters of the ECochG technique.

During lectures Bill remembers Michel Portmann saying, 'Here are the two ears ...' He would then proceed to draw the internal details of the left ear with his left hand while simultaneously drawing the right ear with his right hand. When Bill visited the surgical unit of the University Hospital Pellegrin, he observed that Michel was also able to perform operations on the tiny bones inside the ear, called the ossicles, with both hands simultaneously. Bill remembers that Michel, who was about twenty years his senior, was always very generous with his time. 'He was a beautiful surgeon and a beautiful man.'

Bill also had the good fortune of meeting Michel's wife, Claudine Portmann, a tireless fighter for children with hearing disabilities, who had helped to establish the first Hearing and Language Centre in the Bordeaux region.[4] They had two daughters, Annie and Nathalie, and a son, Didier, who would one day occupy a senior leadership role at the institute.

Bill met quite a few Americans on the course, including Derald Brackmann, who was staying in a hotel across the road from the institute. Their career paths would cross several times in the years ahead but Bill remembers that they first met over lunch in Bordeaux.

Having lunch is an important daily ritual for the French, which should not be forsaken even for a serious course about medicine and electrophysiology. Bill recalls, 'We used to go off and have a full-blown meal at lunchtime and then we would all come back and fall asleep. We went to little restaurants all around Bordeaux.' The weather was warm, so the course participants sat outside the cafés, and the waiters brought out their food, coffee and carafes of wine. Bill says the English didn't yet go in for garlicky food and he remembers reeking for hours after ordering *escargot* from the menu. The wines were always from Bordeaux because the Portmann family were great promoters of their regional wines and even had their own vineyard in a subregion between the Garonne and Dordogne rivers called *Entre-Deux-Mers*.

The first of Bill and Alex's houseguests were Peter and Elvira Carr, who enjoyed spending time with their small grandchildren, Laura and Hugh. The track to the beach from the villa was an incline of about 600 metres through a forest of maritime pine trees which had a spongy carpet of pine needles over an underlay of sand. Bill remembers taking Alex's father with them one day, but he had difficulty with the walk due to his terrible emphysema. When the family reached the end of the forest track they discovered that, as on other European beaches, many of the women were topless.

Within a couple of weeks, other guests started to arrive, including Astrid and John Gibson from Exeter and their daughters Tina and Gay. 'We squeezed them all in,' says Bill with a smile. His sister and brother-in-law, Eleanor and Richard Marshall, came with their three daughters but stayed in another house nearby. At lunchtime they all convened in a tent in the backyard of Bill and Alex's villa to enjoy local seafood from the Bay of Arcachon.

This bay is also known for the largest of its white sand dunes, *La Grande Dune*, which rises more than a hundred metres above sea level. Bill says the reward for climbing the steps carved into the side of this huge sand dune is the view from the top of the French–Atlantic coastline, which stretches nearly all the way down to Spain.

By the end of the holiday they had all roasted themselves until they were 'brown as berries'. Bill recalls that Peter Carr was able to walk each day through the pine forest to the beach and seemed in better health than he had been for years. Bill would never forget the two months he spent in Bordeaux, participating in an electrophysiology course while sampling some of this region's excellent red wines. What he learned in this course and the people he met would later open doors and change the direction of his life in the most unexpected of ways.

* * *

Bill had not worked on the south side of the river Thames until he became a research registrar for Ellis Douek at Guy's Hospital. This beautiful brick and stone hospital, established in 1726, is in the very centre of old London, only a block back from the London Bridge and the Globe Theatre. Just around the bend of the river and directly opposite the Houses of Parliament is St Thomas's Hospital, which Bill visited to see where his sister Eleanor had once worked as a physiotherapist and his father undertook his medical training.

About 80 per cent of Bill's time was occupied with original research towards his MD, and he comments that, 'The doctorate of medicine I did with Ellis Douek at Guy's Hospital was an optional extra that seemed like a good idea at the time. Not many people had this additional degree, so it potentially allowed me to stand out from the crowd.'

The remaining 20 per cent of Bill's time comprised clinical work, including a hearing clinic. About half the children Bill saw in the clinic with significant hearing loss had been deafened by German measles. 'I saw hundreds of these cases. Before children were given the MMR [measles, mumps and rubella] vaccine, German measles was the most common cause of deafness in children.' He explains that another cause of deafness that is also seldom seen today is Rhesus incompatibility. 'RH negative mothers make antibodies against their Rh positive babies and those antibodies can cross the placenta and destroy the hearing of the baby.' He adds that a jaundiced appearance can be a sign of this incompatibility in a newborn and an indication to the nurse or doctor that the baby requires a hearing test.

Hearing is a subjective sensation and Bill remembers that either he or the midwives would crinkle some greaseproof paper to see if a baby turned towards 'the scratchy sound'. However, Bill's youngest patients were not always cooperative or able to communicate what they could hear. For his MD project, Bill developed a simple hearing test which involved the recording of a muscle twitch behind a child's ears in response to a sound. The Preyer reflex, as this twitch is called, is something that humans are no longer aware of, but it is the same response that allows animals such as deer to prick up their ears when they hear a sound. Bill refined the methods employed by Bickford and his co-workers at the University of California during the 1960s[5] to create a new hearing test which could be performed while a child is awake.

In a glossy reprint of Bill's study on fifty-two children aged between five months and eleven years,[6] there is a photo of a mother wearing a striped mini-dress and knee-high boots with a fair-haired toddler sitting on her lap. Bill comments, 'That's Hugh. He was a cute little boy. Alex was holding him on her lap for the photo because someone had to hold the child still while I was doing the test.'

Alex had her hands full these days with four-year-old Laura, two-year-old Hugh and a baby, Gemma, who Bill says, 'was fair like her sister, but had a rounder face'. When Bill returned home from the hospital in the evenings he read stories and poetry to the children, just as his father had once done for him and his siblings. Laura and Hugh adored the Hilaire Belloc poem 'Jim: who ran away from his nurse and was eaten by a lion'. When Bill read the line, 'With open jaws, a lion sprang, and hungrily began to eat', they sprang into the air and let out a lion's roar.

One night Bill and Alex heard what sounded like a baby's crying coming from the front of the house. They looked under their Cortina station wagon to find two abandoned tabby kittens, which they adopted and named Pauline and Barbara. With three children and two cats, the Gibson family was running out of space in their tiny attached house in Highgate.

There were other young families in Claremont Road and the Gibsons also socialised with families in the area including Bill's friend from the Middlesex Hospital, John Graham. John and his wife Sandy lived at the top of the Highgate Hill, which Bill describes as 'the more up-market side of the Archway Road'. At this stage the Grahams had one son, Alastair, who was a couple of years older than Laura, and they would later have two more children in quick succession.

Bill went to talks with John at various hospitals, including the Royal Ear Hospital, which was just around the corner from the Middlesex Hospital. John introduced Bill to the head of the department, Graham Fraser, who asked if he would like to give a presentation about his hearing test for babies. In his talk, Bill explained that he placed an electrode behind the ear of the baby and made a clicking sound. 'If the child can hear, a message is sent to the brainstem, which sends a message back to these central muscles.' Bill referred to these measurements of a muscle response as postauricular myogenic evoked potentials because the 'myo' prefix comes from the Latin word for muscle. He comments, 'If the muscles behind the ear don't twitch, the baby might be deaf'.

Graham Fraser was interested in finding a way to diagnose deafness in babies and thought the equipment Bill had devised would work well in a clinical setting. The Medical Physics Department, which was next door to the Royal Ear Hospital, constructed a device to measure this muscle reflex, which was housed in a white metal box and called 'PAM 1'.[7] Several hundred of these white boxes were sold, resulting in the detection of deafness in a number of children at an early age. However, measurements of this muscle reflex were eventually superseded by responses to sounds from other nearby structures – such as the brainstem and/or the vestibular system, which is responsible for our sense of balance.

* * *

During the year he spent at Guy's Hospital, Bill found Ellis Douek to be a most 'personable' boss. He invited Bill to his family home in the northern London suburb of Hampstead and shared details of his life growing up by the river Nile in Egypt before moving to London to undertake his medical degree. Douek also told Bill about a proud moment from early in his medical career, while he was working in the American Hospital in Paris during the 1960s. 'Ellis told me he had stayed up all night with the French cabaret singer Edith Piaf, who was so thin that he struggled to put the drip up her veins.'

Douek was not only personable but very generous. He paid for Bill and an engineer, Keith Humphries, to fly with him to Bordeaux, where they attended a conference with some of the leading figures in the field of electrophysiology. When this same international study group had met in Vienna two years before, they had come up with 'electric response audiometry', or ERA, as a blanket term to describe a range of tests used for measuring bioelectric hearing responses. Over the next decade Bill would become an expert in ERA and write a book on the subject.

The guest of honour and chairman of the International ERA Study Group in Bordeaux was the retired American professor, Hallowell Davis, who is widely acknowledged as the father of electrophysiology. He even coined the term 'audiology' for a new discipline which involved 'the science of hearing'.[8] Davis was interested in the basic physiology of the inner ear and elucidated the way neurological impulses are transmitted from a pea-sized, shell-like structure called the 'cochlea' – which is deeply embedded in the temporal bone of the inner ear – to the brain via the hearing nerves. Davis's clinical research provided the knowledge required for the development of hearing tests based on electrical responses, as well as improved hearing aids and a new device called the cochlear implant.

While Bill was working on his own MD project, he was aware that Ellis Douek was involved in a project to develop a cochlear implant. Through the Voice Clinic Douek ran at Guy's Hospital he had started working with a scientist and voice pitch expert from University College Hospital (UCH), Adrian Fourcin. Douek and Fourcin collaborated on a device which Bill describes as 'extra-cochlear', because it sat on the surface of the cochlea rather than inside, as was the case for later cochlear implants.

Douek's interest in this new field had begun in Paris about a decade before his emotional encounter with Edith Piaf. At seventeen, Douek went with his mother to visit his brother in a Parisian hospital. His brother's surgeon, Roger Maspétiol, took Douek to meet a teenage Vietnamese girl he had operated on. She had a copper wire peeping out from the bandages around her head and Douek recalls that a French professor was calling out to her in exaggerated tones, 'Allo, allo'.

Douek thinks this professor was almost certainly André Djourno of the Faculté de Médecine at the University of Paris who, together with the French ear surgeon Charles Eyriès, developed the world's first cochlear implant.[9] The Vietnamese girl was the second patient to receive their device. The first recipient said he could hear cricket-like sounds and simple words such as 'mama', 'papa' and 'allo'. Djourno and Eyriès published their findings in the 1957 edition of the French journal *Presse Médicale* and Eyriès subsequently withdrew from the project.[10] Two years after this publication, Djourno also decided to abandon the cochlear implant project. A patient of the American otolaryngologist William House brought him a translation of an article about the French implants and he pursued the idea himself in 1961 with an engineer named Doyle.[11]

There was some progress over the next decade with cochlear implants made by several groups in America and Europe, including a former student of Eyriès, Claude-Henri Chouard. However, Bill remembers there being a 'scientific pushback' by some leading physiologists, including Nelson Kiang from Harvard in the US, who cautioned against using cochlear implants in humans until animal studies had proven them to be safe.

Then in 1973, while Bill was working at Guy's Hospital, William House and a different engineer, Jack Urban, 'broke rank' by publishing a paper describing further implant operations on three patients. The paper, published in the *Annals of Otology,* described the use of an insulated 'platinum wire' device which was inserted into the cochlea.[12] In his clipping file Bill also has an article published in the *National Times* in July 1973, which mentions an implant operation on a young British woman.[13] This operation, using the same platinum wire device, was performed by William House and Derald Brackmann, who Bill had met the previous year at the Institut Georges Portmann in Bordeaux.

As an ENT surgeon, Bill already had at his disposal the stapedectomy operation, which had proven to be very effective for the treatment of 'conductive deafness'. He was now excited about the prospect of having an implantable device for use in patients who suffered from 'sensory deafness', which results from damage to the thousands of tiny sensory hair cells lining the fluid-filled cochlea. There was currently very little that could be done for these patients if hearing aids provided no benefit.

The field was now wide open for groups across the world to progress their plans for an implanted cochlear device. Some of the front-runners Bill read about in the medical press were Ingeborg Hochmair and her husband Erwin Hochmair, from a team led by Kurt Burian at the Technical University of Vienna, and a team led by Graeme Clark at the University of Melbourne. Just as the French paper had provided the inspiration for William House, it was a paper by Blair Simmons from Stanford University that had inspired Graeme Clark to make 'a contribution' to this burgeoning field.[14]

Bill's good friend John Graham would later become very interested in the origins of the cochlear implant story, particularly the early French chapter, which remained largely unknown for several decades. He believes that the realisation of a workable cochlear implant came about through the efforts of scientists in several countries over a number of years, which at a certain stage 'achieved synchrony'.[15]

Bill recalls that Ellis Douek and Adrian Fourcin continued to work on their cochlear device in the years ahead, but like many groups, never reached the stage of commercialisation involving human trials. However, they received a standing ovation when they first presented a talk on their extra-cochlear device at the Otology Section of the Royal Society of Medicine.

Bill considers that the presentation on his MD project and the other talks he gave at the Royal Society of Medicine were helpful in raising his profile with colleagues within his own specialisation. They also undoubtedly assisted him in securing an interview for a senior registrar's position at the prestigious London Hospital, located in the not so salubrious Whitechapel district. This position was the last rung of the career ladder he needed to climb to be accredited by the Royal College of Surgeons as having attained 'higher surgical standing' and thus be able to apply for a coveted consultant ENT position. Fortunately for Bill, his interview at the London Hospital turned out to be one of the easiest he ever attended.

CHAPTER 6

The London Triumvirate

Every month another clinical paper with our three names at the top appeared in a respected medical journal. It caused quite a stir in ENT circles and colleagues started calling us 'The London Triumvirate'.

David Moffat, emeritus consultant
in neuro-otology, Addenbrookes
Hospital, Cambridge

While Bill Gibson waited nervously for his name to be called in a room at the back of the London Hospital, commonly known as The London, he struck up a conversation with another candidate for the senior registrar's position. This other candidate sounded annoyed when he remarked, 'I don't know why I've wasted my time coming all this way. I've been told that some fellow named Gibson is going to get the job.'

There was nothing arduous about Bill's interview. One of the four people on the interview panel — which included three senior ENT consultants and a representative from the hospital administration – simply asked some questions such as, 'Why do you want the job?' Senior registrars from the Department of Otolaryngology were attached on a rotational basis to the same three ENT consultants: Andrew Morrison, John Booth and Peter McKelvie. Of the three, Bill had the greatest rapport with Andrew Morrison, because they shared an interest in the study of ears (otology).

One day as Bill and his new boss were walking together through the main hospital building, which faces Whitechapel Road in Whitechapel, Andrew Morrison pointed to the apex of a staircase spiralling upward and exclaimed, 'That's where they took Joseph Merrick when he first arrived at this hospital in 1886!' The Elephant Man, as Merrick is better known, is one of the hospital's most iconic patients and Bill would sometimes go down to the Hospital Museum, located in the crypt of St Philip's church, to see the exhibit featuring Merrick's travelling cloak and cap, along with his grossly disfigured skeleton.[1]

The other exhibit that intrigued Bill related to Jack the Ripper, whose identity has never been determined. This infamous 19th-century murderer deposited the bodies of at least five prostitutes around the streets of Whitechapel, which has never lost its sinister reputation. 'The Ripper removed the kidney from one victim and the uterus from another. It seemed likely that he was someone with very good surgical skills. The consultants were concerned that he had formerly been a surgeon at The London.'

It was from Andrew Morrison and a neurosurgeon, Tom King, that Bill learnt how to remove a tumour from the hearing nerve known as an acoustic neuroma. They co-authored a paper on this surgical procedure, entitled 'Tumours of the eighth cranial nerve', for the *British Journal of Hospital Medicine*,[2] which was translated the following year into Spanish.

Between his busy operating schedules and outpatient clinics, Bill also needed to ensure he set aside sufficient time for his electrophysiology work. Andrew Morrison encouraged him to continue with this important research activity and even introduced him to a mentor named Harry Beagley, who Bill considered to be 'the leading guy in England in this kind of testing'. Bill worked for Harry a half-day per week as an honorary senior registrar at one of the two branches of the Royal National Throat, Nose and Ear Hospital. This branch, in Gray's Inn Road, would become one of the largest ENT hospitals in the world.[3] It is still referred to today as 'Gray's Inn Road', and when Bill worked there it was the sister hospital of 'Golden Square' in Soho, which was later converted into a hotel.

This unpaid research position meant that Bill was able to test the hearing of children in the paediatric wards and clinics conducted at the Nuffield Centre, named after William Morris, who founded Morris Motors and was raised to the peerage as Lord Nuffield. It had already been shown that tests based on electrical responses such as electrocochleography (ECochG) could be used as a way of measuring hearing. However, Bill and Beagley hoped this test could be used to diagnose conditions such as Menière's disease and acoustic neuromas. They postulated that ECochGs would one day prove as useful to otologists as the electrocardiogram (EEG) was to cardiologists.[4]

Bill held Beagley in the highest regard, but found this New Zealander to be very reclusive. 'Harry was a nice man but he was so private that you couldn't really get to know him. I never met his family or went out for a drink with him. If we went to a conference, he wouldn't even go to the conference dinners.'

When Beagley was invited to present a paper at the inaugural meeting on Evoked Potentials in Seville, he asked his young protégé to go in his place and Bill jumped at the opportunity. 'I was just a young fella and everything was laid on for free. I remember eating *all* this crayfish.' When Bill had recovered sufficiently from a bout of food poisoning, he travelled to the ski slopes of the Sierra Nevada, in the south-east of Spain. He says, with a cheeky grin, 'I was quite put out, because the King of Spain decided to go skiing the same day. Every time I tried to ski, they'd closed the slope. I thought that was a bit rude, when someone had come all the way from England to ski in their country.'

* * *

In the mid-1970s Bill enjoyed two family reunions in Dawlish. The first was for the joint christening of his daughter Gemma and Bob's daughter Jenny in July 1974, when the girls were about ten months and six months respectively. For the second reunion, during the summer of 1975, Bill's sister Kathy and brother-in-law Martin came from Canada and brought their three daughters, Penny, Nikki and Kelsey. Bill remembers these holidays as special times.

Later in the same school holidays of 1975 Bill and his family went away with their neighbours from Claremont Road to a remote part of Scotland, about 200 miles north-west of Glasgow. They stayed in rustic, white-washed cottages in *Monarch of the Glen*–style countryside, complete with fast-moving streams and gorse-covered hills. Bill took a photo of Laura and Hugh in front of a mob of Highland sheep and recalls that Gemma, not quite two, was already talking and keen to keep up with her older brother and sister. A highlight of the holiday was a fresh salmon picnic on board the boat of the estate's laird, Johnny Noble, who wore a green woollen tam o' shanter. Even though it was August and theoretically summer, Bill remembers there being a chill in the air.

One Saturday morning, not long after returning from Scotland, Bill went to check on his patients at The London, as he usually did, and decided to take Laura and Hugh with him. Their neighbours from Claremont Road asked if Gemma would like to spend the morning with their two little girls.

On his way back from The London, Bill saw his neighbours' car pulled over at the side of the road, with the three little girls sitting in the back. They had run out of petrol, so Bill grabbed a jerrycan from his boot and told Laura and Hugh to wait in the car. While filling his neighbours' car with petrol, he didn't notice that Gemma had climbed out of the car. Bill heard the screeching of brakes but didn't see the moment of impact when Gemma was run over. Afterwards he did everything possible to breathe life into his tiny daughter, but it was too late.

He remembers the details of that Saturday with clarity but the following days and weeks are 'just a blur'. When Bill returned to work, he knew straight away that it was too soon. If a patient was complaining about their tinnitus, or some other problem, he would be thinking, 'What about losing your life when you're only two years old?'

Bill and Alex had two raised clay reliefs crafted of their daughter's face with 'Gemma' written underneath. The better of the two firings still hangs on the wall of the children's waiting room at the Nuffield Centre at Gray's Inn Road, where Bill tested children's hearing with Harry Beagley. When colleagues and friends asked if Bill had set up a fund in Gemma's honour, he would tell them, 'Give the money to the Nuffield for the deaf children'.

Bill's clinical research activities naturally went quiet for a while, but one evening he thought of something quiet and solitary he could do while he was grieving for his daughter. He knew several people who had turned their MD theses into books, and electrophysiological testing of the ear was a new field in which few, if any, books had yet been written. There were two publishers among the group of parents Bill and Alex knew from Laura and Hugh's primary school in Highgate, St Michael's Church of England. One of them, Tim Rix, worked for an educational publisher, Longmans (known today as

Pearsons). Rix thought Bill's idea for a book on clinical testing would be ideally suited to the medical division of Longman's, Churchill Livingstone.

Essentials of Clinical Electric Response Audiometry would not be published for another couple of years, but in the acknowledgments section Bill paid tribute to Alex and his children, who, he wrote, 'have provided the atmosphere of love which has kept me going during the many hours of writing'. Only those closest to Bill would realise the significance of these words, and of the simple dedication printed opposite the book's title: 'To Gemma'.

* * *

Two of Bill's colleagues from The London supported him through this difficult period and became good friends. The first of these was a Scotsman, Richard Ramsden, who had studied medicine at Scotland's oldest university, St Andrew's, but decided to complete his post-qualification medical training in London. A year younger than Bill and of a similar average height, Richard has thick wavy hair, heavy-framed glasses and a cheerful demeanour.

Bill and Richard were soon joined by David Moffat, a registrar in the Otolaryngology Department of The London. David is three years younger than Bill and Richard, so they referred to him as 'Boy Moffat' or just 'the boy'. These were good descriptors for this tall, lanky young man with fair hair and a moustache. It was ultimately a shared wit and intelligence which drew the three of them together. Richard describes it as 'an ability to bounce off each other's jokes with a witty repartee and be able to see the humorous side of a situation'. David says that *badinage* is the French term for the friendly banter they shared. Despite the age gap, David remembers Bill and Richard being extremely kind and including him in all their socialising and research.

This included the occasional game of golf, and also regular drinks with other colleagues at the Grave Maurice, a pub on Whitechapel Road directly opposite the front entrance to The London. There was a table in the dark and dingy bar of this pub permanently reserved for the infamous Kray Brothers, and an old man commented to Bill one day, 'There will be no justice in the East End now that the Kray Brothers have been put away.' Bill thinks he was probably referring to the little old ladies who could not afford their rent and had no one to protect them now from greedy, heartless landlords.

Richard and David were impressed by the knowledge of electrophysiology Bill had gained from his time at the Institut Georges Portmann and they knew about his passion for finding a cure for Menière's disease. During the early days of his search for a cure Bill could sometimes think of nothing else for hours on end. David cites the example of the day he rang Bill to ask what time he would like to be picked up for a clinical meeting. After a prolonged silence he enquired, 'Are you still there?', to which Bill replied, 'I might have the answer to Menière's disease! I was thinking about it while I was lying in the bath last night.'

As a continuation of the electrocochleography work he had already done with Harry Beagley, Bill tested a series of patients who had no known cause of Menière's disease but suffered from the classic triad of symptoms: fluctuating hearing loss, episodes of vertigo and tinnitus. Much to the surprise of Bill and his two colleagues from The London, they found a recognisable abnormality in the ECochGs of 65 per cent of the patients they tested. They were able to consistently record this abnormality, which they described as 'wide and distorted waveforms' on the purple ink traces of the ECochG printout. The most likely explanation for these altered waveforms was the presence of increased levels of endolymphatic fluid in the inner ears of the Menière's patients, due to a condition called endolymphatic hydrops. These waveforms differed from those of healthy patients, so it could be used as a diagnostic test and also a predictor for which patients would benefit from surgery to drain their endolymphatic sac.

The paper on the diagnosis and management of Menière's disease Bill published in the *International Journal of Audiology*, with Ramsden and Moffat as his co-authors, is undoubtedly the most important paper he has written.[5] Just as a legal precedent can be quoted for time immemorial, this paper is still being quoted in the medical literature today, nearly forty years later. 'Nobody had ever showed the distorted waveforms before, so it was my claim to fame,' says Bill, smiling broadly. 'Obviously, it would have been nice if there had also been a cure but we were adding to our knowledge about Menière's disease all the time.'

In October 1976, Bill presented these important findings at the 13th International Congress of Audiology at the Palazzo dei Congressi, on via Valfonda, in Florence. His presentation was late on the last day of the conference and he notes that 'Ironically, there was hardly a soul around to hear it'.

During the same year, he was invited by Michel Portmann to an anniversary celebration for the Institut Georges Portmann and its Foundation. During his visit to Bordeaux, Bill literally bumped into a more senior ENT surgeon from Australia named Barry Scrivener, who was undertaking a one-year Fellowship at the institute. Scrivener must have seen something promising in Bill because as part of their ongoing correspondence he said that he would keep him in mind as a presenter for future ENT courses at the University of Sydney.

Between conferences, Bill always made sure to be home for his children's birthday parties. He enjoys dressing up and one year he wore a peaked cap, a shaggy 'onesie' and a pointy nose made out of cardboard. 'I was one of the Wombles of Wimbledon Common,' says Bill, referring to a stop-motion children's television show, *The*

Wombles, which aired in the mornings on the BBC. Bill's party tricks included balancing a chair on his chin and placing a pea in one ear and then pretending to take it out from his other ear. Once, when one of the peas became stuck and Bill used a 'looped-over paper clip to wiggle it out', some blood trickled out from his ear. Alex suggested that he present himself at The London, but Bill was worried that Ramsden or Moffat might be on duty and comments, 'I would never have heard the end of it'.

These two friends had formed the opinion early on that Bill was 'a brilliant guy, but the archetypal absent-minded professor'. Richard can recall the time that Bill was invited to give a lecture 'somewhere in Scotland' and said to him, 'I think the place starts with the letter G'. A few weeks later Richard received a long-distance call from Bill, saying, 'I'm here. The meeting is in Glasgow, but I'm a week early. Can you please do my clinics for me?' David comments that this was before Alex became Bill's medical secretary. 'The only reason Bill gets anywhere is because of Alex. She's the power behind the throne.'

* * *

The three colleagues and their wives met regularly for dinner parties. They were not your regular evening get-togethers, because after dinner the husbands adjourned to another room to write a research paper. During their first few of these writing sessions, they drank red wine with dinner but it quickly became apparent to Bill that they were not very productive if they 'hit the wine too early'.

The various stages of planning, clinical work and writing up of an academic paper can take many months, sometimes years. Bill and his two colleagues devised a plan whereby they could speed up this process by meeting three times a month. The first meeting was to decide on a new research angle; the second was to write a rough draft; and the third meeting was to decide if the paper was acceptable for submission. Using this formula, they set out to publish a clinical paper every month for twelve months in a row so their names would be in print for a whole year. For the kind of peer-reviewed medical journals they wished to target, each paper would need to be approved by not only the journal editor but at least two reviewers.

The wide and distorted waveforms that Bill and his colleagues had already demonstrated in the ECochGs of Menière's patients could be consistently recorded at intervals of less than a minute apart, so this test could be used to monitor the effects of pharmacological agents upon the human cochlea. Bill will always remember the 'start of their run' being a paper on the effects of a vasodilatory drug, naftidrofuryl, on Menière's patients.[6] Most of the patients in the study noted an increase in their hearing for at least an hour after the infusion of naftidrofuryl into their ears but the benefits were not long-lasting enough for it to be recommended as a treatment. As the first author of this paper Bill presented their findings on 3 December 1976 in the Otology Section at the Royal Society of Medicine.

Setting out to host and/or attend something like thirty-six dinner parties in one year might seem a daunting prospect for some people but not these three fun-loving couples. Bill comments, 'We were good friends who were all fired up and writing papers together'. Richard's former wife, Wendy, has a First-class Honours degree in English from St Andrew's and offered to proofread their clinical papers. She also extended this same offer to Bill for his book.

Over the previous couple of years Bill's book had become a 200-plus-page treatise on everything to do with electric response audiometry. Bill is fascinated by medical history so he naturally included a discussion of one of the pioneers in the field, Luigi Galvani, who had discovered the electrical activity of biological tissue 200 years earlier.

The publisher at the medical division of Longmans wrote to inform Bill that they had secured someone well known in the field of electrical testing to write the foreword for his book. Bob Ruben, a professor at the Albert Einstein College of Medicine in New York, lived in the Bronx, which was known at this time for the gangs ruling its streets. When Bill stayed with Ruben to discuss the contents of his book, he remembers that the two of them drove around with locked car doors in case of an armed hold-up.

Another American who became very interested in Bill's electrophysiology studies was Kaufman 'Irv' Arenberg, who was the assistant professor of surgery in the Division of Otolaryngology at the University of Wisconsin. When he visited England, Arenberg caused murmurs among the conservative ENT consultants at The London with his long sideburns, moustache and flamboyant, 1970s style of dress. This first introduction at the hospital led to future research collaborations between Bill and Arenberg, including clinical meetings in Denver, Colorado, where this American colleague later settled.

Bill was aware that American ENT specialists had expressed concerns about the ECochG test because it involved the surgeon inserting a long, fine needle through the 'tympanic membrane' – the scientific name for the ear drum between the outer and middle ear. The US Food and Drug Administration (FDA) considered there was a possibility that the procedure might cause pain or medical complications for the patient.[7]

In Bill's experience, no patient had ever asked him 'to abandon the procedure or refused to have the second ear tested'.[8] When Bill performed an ECochG on a child he always did it under a general anaesthetic to keep them sufficiently still during the testing. Adults are tested while they are awake and to make them more comfortable Richard Ramsden came up with the idea of spraying the tympanic membrane with a topical anaesthetic called Cetacaine.

Richard was the first author of this paper, which added to their prolific publishing *oeuvre*.[9]

During a twelve-month period in 1977 and 1978, the *Journal of Laryngology and Otology* regularly published articles under the by-line of Gibson, Ramsden and Moffat, in varying order of names. Sometimes there were additional authors, including Bill's friend from the Middlesex Hospital, John Graham, who they had invited to join them for dinner one night when he had an idea for a paper on sudden hearing loss.[10]

They published some of their findings in different medical journals, for example a paper with Ramsden as first author in the *Annals of Otology, Rhinology and Laryngology*, which described a study of patients with hearing loss and syphilis.[11] Moffat was the first author of a paper published in *Acta Oto-Laryngologica* which described the effects of infusing glycerol into the ear before performing an ECochG on patients with Menière's disease.[12] The glycerol had a dehydrating effect on the ears of the Menière's patients, but not on those of healthy subjects, and made a definitive diagnosis of the disease more likely.

Like Bill's paper on the wide and distorted waveforms, Moffat's glycerol dehydration paper is still being quoted in the literature today. Moffat recalls, 'We were right at the forefront of electrophysiology research so it was an exciting period. Every month another clinical paper with our three names at the top appeared in a respected medical journal. It caused quite a stir in ENT circles and colleagues started calling us "The London Triumvirate". This translates as three people who succeed at something such as politics, sport or in this case medical research.'

Despite their elevated standing in the world of medical research, the three friends still delighted in 'taking the mickey' out of each other. Bill will never forget the time he returned to The London at the end of a long summer break to find a sign

Ramsden and Moffat had tacked to the side of his cubicle saying, 'Gone for good'.

* * *

Bill had taken his family down to Dawlish for what would be their last holiday in his childhood home. When Bill's father decided to retire as a general practitioner, it seemed like a good time to move out of Whickham Lodge, with its eight bedrooms and two staircases, which was a great relief to his mother. His parents were about to move into a three-bedroom cottage at the end of their gravel driveway, called Whickham Cottage, and his mother was in a mad frenzy of 'chucking out', as Bill called it.

'Alex and I are real hoarders, but mum was more prone to say "No use now" and throw things away. Every time I came home from medical school she had chucked something away.' Years before, Jane had taken her father's lovely old radios to the rubbish dump and now Bill discovered that she had given her father's black onyx carriage clock to the local old people's home. He said to her, 'Oh, no. I want that back', and fortunately the staff at the home were sympathetic. Bill installed the clock, with the little plaque on the front engraved with 'Charles Rea Esq BA BSc, 1893', on the mantlepiece of his new family home in London.

The four-storey home Bill and Alex purchased at 75 Onslow Gardens, Muswell Hill, had black Tudor details on the white-painted brickwork. It was the last in a row of early Victorian terrace houses which swept in a gentle curve all the way back to the beginning of their road. It was much bigger than their previous home, about a mile away in Claremont Road, and Bill says that at nearly £50000, 'Its price tag was much bigger too'.

The Gibson family now had commanding views of London and the huge crystal structure known as Alexandra Palace, or 'Ally

Pally', from which the BBC broadcast their programs. From their top-floor windows at night the lights of London were like a sparkling wonderland. It was in this home that Bill and his family celebrated Queen Elizabeth II's Silver Jubilee on 7 June 1977 with a street party. It was a wonderful excuse to meet their neighbours, including Heinz Wolff, the professor of psychiatry from the Middlesex Hospital who had allowed Bill and his friend John Graham to sit in on his psychotherapy sessions.

When Bill was later a professor himself and had his own trainee surgeons, some of them would ask, 'Who was driving this incredible publishing period? Was it you or Ramsden?' The three close friends had missed by one month their goal of having their names appear in a medical journal every month for a year. Perhaps it was Bill who egged the others on, but in the end it was a group effort. It also happened at a juncture in history when electrical testing of the inner ear was at the forefront of the medical world's knowledge and imagination. In fact, Bill thinks of the 1970s as 'the golden age of electrocochleography'. Richard Ramsden agrees that the timing was an important factor and quotes from a speech made by Brutus in Shakespeare's *Julius Caesar*:

> There is a tide in the affairs of men,
> Which, taken at the flood, leads on to fortune;
> Omitted, all the voyage of their life
> Is bound in shallows and in the miseries.

Ramsden comments, 'If you follow my metaphor, we were able to surf that flood.'

The never-to-be repeated run of articles authored by the three colleagues from The London proved helpful for all of their careers. Before the eleventh paper was even published Bill had been offered a consultant's post at Queen's Square in London, and Richard

Ramsden's consultant appointment at the Royal Manchester Infirmary followed the next year. David Moffat stayed on at The London as a senior registrar and a couple of years later became a consultant in neuro-otology – a subspecialty of ENT concerned with neurological diseases of the ears – and skull base surgery at Addenbrooke's Hospital in Cambridge.

At a dinner party to celebrate Bill's appointment as a consultant, the three couples took humorous photos of each other in a variety of poses. Bill can be seen in one photo looking suave in a blue suit, holding a slim cigar. The friends would remain close, despite living in different locations, and The London Triumvirate would all go on to become important men in their respective careers.

CHAPTER 7

A major decision

It was a major decision, because Alex
and I had kids still in school and both
sets of parents alive. We felt terrible
because we knew we'd be taking their
grandchildren away from them.

Bill Gibson

In September 1977 Bill Gibson started work as a consultant ENT
surgeon at Queen Square, so called because of its location in one
of London's garden squares. 'Its correct title was the National
Hospital for Nervous Diseases', says Bill, smiling as he adds, 'They
later changed its name because it sounded as if someone had to be
nervous or anxious to be a patient. It is actually the leading neurology hospital in England and neurologists come from all around the
world to gain clinical experience there.'

During the seven years Bill worked at Queen Square he met
quite a few Australians and would later wonder if this was a sign.
His first impression of Michael Halmagyi was 'the strange Australian
with no money'. The lack of funds became obvious the evening
Michael and Susan Halmagyi invited Bill and Alex, along with

another couple from the hospital, to their flat for dinner and they all had to sit on packing cases. Despite being a fully qualified neurologist, Michael was supporting a family of five in London on a neuro-otology fellow's wage of £6000 per year.

In a professional relationship that has continued to this day, the only clinical paper they wrote together at Queen Square was a case study of a woman who displayed an unusual cluster of symptoms for a few weeks after Bill had performed a stapedectomy operation on her left ear. During this period, Bill noticed that her eyes had a 'screwed-up' orientation and that her head and body both tilted to the left. Halmagyi postulated that one of her otolith organs, responsible for maintaining balance, had been affected during her operation. They coined the term 'ocular tilt reaction' for this previously undescribed pattern of responses.[1] Like Bill's important distorted waveforms ECochG paper, this observation was a chance discovery, with Halmagyi noting that 'Everything, in hindsight, is elementary'.

The Halmagyis' flat in Highgate was not far from where Bill and Alex lived in Muswell Hill. On a hunch that his colleague was not well, Michael called in to see Bill one weekend and made a provisional diagnosis of pneumonia. After having a chest X-ray Bill rang his father to tell him he had lobar pneumonia. John was terribly worried that Bill might have allowed the pneumonia to progress to the 'red hepatisation' stage, where a person's lungs become meaty and airless. Bill explains that 'In Victorian times people suffered a crisis and either lived or died. But fortunately, we have antibiotics now.'

When the NHS was first introduced, Bill's father told him that consultant surgeons were 'bribed with gold'. Now Bill was employed by the NHS in this same role. In what may seem like an unusual workplace arrangement, he was required to devote nine-elevenths of his working week to treating public patients. Bill conducted these sessions at both Queen Square and University College Hospital, where he obtained a paid locum consultant's position because the previous consultant had a drinking problem.

Even though Bill inherited some patients at Queen Square from his predecessors, Spencer Harrison and Sir Terence Cawthorne, it took a while for his sessions to fill up so he had a short period of time to 'catch his breath' and play a little golf. One of the social contacts Bill made through his children's primary school in Highgate was Gerry Sinstadt, a well-known football commentator for Granada Television. Most Tuesday mornings they played eighteen holes at the Highgate Golf Club, and Bill notes that 'Fortunately, we were as hopeless at golf as each other'.

For the other two-elevenths of his working week, Bill was permitted to see private patients in some consulting rooms at Queen Square. He conducted the electrophysiological testing on these patients at the London Otological Centre in Cavendish Street, Marylebone. The audiologists at this centre performed behavioural tests on children to assess their hearing, and those found to be 'hyperkinetic' and/or difficult to manage were referred to Bill so that he could perform electrophysiological testing under a general anaesthetic.

Nearly all the children referred to the centre came from overseas, including many from Middle Eastern countries such as Saudi Arabia. Bill thought the boys he tested who were found to be deaf would probably be cared for and put into a home, but he worried that a bad prognosis might mean 'curtains for the girls'. Along with two colleagues from the London Otological Centre, Bill tested nearly one-hundred children using brain stem potentials and electrocochleography and found the latter test to be both the quickest to perform and the easiest to interpret.[2]

Bill used these same electrophysiology tests to conduct research with his colleagues at the Hearing and Balance Unit at Queen

Square. He wrote quite a few papers with an Indian PhD scientist named Deepak Prasher and together they located small brain lesions or plaques on the brainstem that are characteristic of patients with multiple sclerosis (MS).[3] The famous English cellist Jacqueline du Pré was already wheelchair-bound when she made an appointment at Queen Square and Bill was able to demonstrate abnormalities typical of MS in her brainstem potentials.

One of the most interesting electrocochleography papers Bill wrote at this time was co-authored with a senior registrar from the Royal Free Hospital, Rob Black, an Australian who would later establish a successful ENT practice on Queensland's Gold Coast. The idea for the paper arose during the three years Bill worked at The London, where he encountered patients in the late stages of syphilis who displayed Menière's-like symptoms, including hearing loss and dizziness. Bill and Rob explored the possible role of a bacterial infection, such as syphilis or yaws – a contagious disease found in tropical countries – as the causative agent in the symptoms of four patients with fluctuating hearing loss who were of West Indian or African extraction.[4] 'You wouldn't expect to see Menière's symptoms in dark-skinned people, but these four patients were the exception,' says Bill, who comments that these findings brought into question long-established beliefs about this disease.

* * *

Menière's can be a grim subject to discuss, so for the presentations Bill gave on this disease in his own department and at other hospitals he used as an icebreaker a Hilaire Belloc poem he could recite by heart, entitled 'The Chief Defect of Henry King'. This poem always produced a few laughs, because it was true that people had been searching for a cure for Menière's disease for over a hundred years:

The Chief Defect of Henry King
Was chewing little bits of String.
At last he swallowed some which tied
Itself in ugly Knots inside.

Physicians of the Utmost Fame
Were called at once; but when they came
They answered, as they took their Fees,
'There is no Cure for this Disease'.

A colleague working in Bill's department, Margaret Dix, was present for these talks. Before World War II, she had been a contemporary of the famous otologist Charles Hallpike. Together they had developed the 'Dix–Hallpike Manoeuvre', which has been used since 1952 as a diagnostic test for a common form of vertigo and dizziness, benign paroxysmal positional vertigo (BPPV).[5] This manoeuvre involves the doctor lowering a patient's head from the upright position towards the examination table while observing their eyes for a rapid flickering behind the eyelids, known as nystagmus.

Bill describes Margaret Dix as 'a lovely lady who was very English and owned about a hundred cats'. He never mentions the disfigurement on one side of her face, which was the result of a bomb blast during World War II. Margaret proposed Bill for membership of the Collegium Oto-Rhino-Laryngologicum Amicitiae Sacrum (CORLAS), which loosely translates as 'a group of sacred friends from the ENT profession'. At thirty-four, Bill was the youngest member to be admitted to CORLAS, which had been founded after World War I to provide a neutral ground for medical discussions.[6]

At his first CORLAS meeting in Budapest, Bill met several 'very high-up' ENT specialists, including Juergen Tonndorf from

Columbia University, who had served as a commander in the German submarine corps during World War II and emigrated to America in 1947.[7] They shared an interest in the basic physiology of the inner ear and Bill had read Tonndorf's papers describing the way sound vibrations from the eardrum are transmitted via three tiny bones – the malleus, incus and stapes – to the cochlea in the inner ear. The CORLAS meeting was held in late 1978, and Bill witnessed the reality of communism in Hungary, including 'huge red stars on the buildings and stores with nothing to buy except buckets and mops'.

Bill recalls that the UK was experiencing its own problems at this time, including crippling strikes by the trade unions. The newly elected British Prime Minister Margaret Thatcher would earn the title 'Iron Lady' for the range of economic and labour issues she tackled. This was also the midway point in a decade of violent Anglo-Irish clashes and Belfast was the worst affected city. During Bill's three-day visit to the Royal Belfast Hospital he saw soldiers guarding bricklayers as they constructed a 500-yard wall around the perimeter of the hospital. 'The wall was to stop the snipers, because the nurses were complaining about all the bullets coming through the windows,' says Bill. His hosts in Belfast – the Irish ENT surgeons Gordon Smyth and Alan Kerr – made sure that nobody shot at him.

Not surprisingly, the Royal Victorian Hospital in Belfast was regarded as one of the leading hospitals in the world for the treatment of gunshot wounds. Back in London, one of the surgeons Bill worked with in the operating theatres, Alan Crockard, came from Belfast and was also an expert at removing bullets from the heads of soldiers. The operations Bill performed with Crockard at a sister hospital of Queen Square, Maida Vale Hospital for Nervous Diseases, involved the removal of benign, slow-growing tumours called acoustic neuromas, which only become dangerous if they are allowed to become large and press on the brainstem. Bill sometimes removed tumours 'as big as tangerines' in gruelling operations lasting up to nine hours; however, with two surgeons in the operating theatre he says it was possible to 'take a break and have a cup of tea'.

Alan Crockard was the first surgeon Bill had encountered who played music in the operating theatre but it was something he also came to enjoy. 'Crockard loved his classical music,' says Bill, who remembers the two of them listening to Mozart sonatas and Verdi's 'Chorus of the Hebrew Slaves' from the opera *Nabucco*. Bill and Alex had their own favourite pieces of classical music, such as Pachelbel's 'Canon', but they preferred the popular music of bands such as the Beatles and the Rolling Stones. Bill had also become a fan of ABBA after seeing their winning song 'Waterloo' telecast live from Brighton in the UK during the 1974 Eurovision song contest.

ABBA hits such as 'Take a Chance on Me' and 'Gimme, Gimme, Gimme' featured on the compilation cassette tapes Bill played as he and his family drove along *L'autoroute du Soleil* – the motorway of the sun – from Lyon to Argelès-sur-Mer on the warm Mediterranean Sea. This French town is located on a wide, sweeping bay overlooking the Pyrenees and for three years in a row Bill's sister Eleanor and her family joined them at a camping ground in this idyllic location.

After a couple of trips to the south of France Bill replaced the family's Renault 4 with an Audi and bought a trailer to store their tent and all the rest of their gear. The final holiday the two families enjoyed together in Argelès-sur-Mer was in 1981 because, as Bill can clearly remember, it was the year 'Prince Charles married Lady Diana'. They decorated their campsite with Union Jack bunting and watched the ceremony huddled around a television which a nice Dutchman, named Jarb, had set up outside his caravan. This was the same year that ten-year-old Hugh Gibson showed promise of having the business acumen of his uncle Bob by purchasing an inflatable boat for 10 francs and selling it for 15 – even with a slow leak.

* * *

Bob Gibson had been living in Australia for nearly a decade, but Bill and his family had still not made it out to visit them. 'My brother was always waxing lyrical about how Australia was such a wonderful country,' says Bill. 'I'd read about the Australian medical scene, but I was intrigued to see what the country was like.' When Barry Scrivener invited Bill to be one of the presenters in a neuro-otology course at the University of Sydney in 1981, Bill said to Alex, 'Perhaps we should go and see for ourselves why Bob and Jan think Australia is so great'.

It rained nearly every day while Bill's family were staying in Sydney and he complained to Bob, 'You told us it would be sunny and nice!' While Laura and Hugh remained with their cousins on Sydney's north shore, Bill and Alex checked in to the Travelodge motel on Missenden Road, Camperdown. This motel is only a few hundred yards from the University of Sydney and its teaching hospital, Royal Prince Alfred Hospital, which is commonly referred to as RPA. Barry Scrivener told Bill that they were trying to establish a Chair of Otolaryngology at the university and to have a think about whether he would like to apply. In a photo of the course leaders, Bill can be seen with Barry Scrivener and Derald Brackman, from the House Ear Institute in Los Angeles.

Bill met several well-qualified and influential Australian ENT surgeons on this first visit to Australia, including John Tonkin from St Vincent's Hospital in Sydney. Tonkin was one of the delegates at a CORLAS meeting Bill attended in San Francisco in 1981. One evening, when the collegium delegates visited the men-only country club Bohemian Grove, John Tonkin introduced Bill to the otolaryngologist Horst Wüllstein, who was the first surgeon to successfully graft a perforated ear drum. Bill was fascinated to discover that several of the leading German ENT surgeons he met at collegium meetings, including Tonndorf and Wüllstein, had held senior military roles during World War II. Bill recalls that during a late-night discussion with John Tonkin and himself over a whisky, Wüllstein was very open in sharing his view that 'The world would have been a far better place if Germany had won the war'.

Bill knew that John Tonkin had performed the first cochlear implant operation in Australia in 1977,[8] using the House Institute's single channel device, and regarded him as the most innovative ENT surgeon in Australia. Barry Scrivener was also very well regarded after deciding to specialise in otology when he returned from his year-long Fellowship at the Institut Georges Portmann in Bordeaux.[9] Scrivener saw private patients in his rooms in Macquarie Street in the Sydney CBD, which is known for its many medical specialists' practices.

Bill had by now acquired his own private rooms in the very medical Wimpole Street in London, where the Royal Society of Medicine is located. As he became more senior, Bill had been able to 'whittle down' his NHS obligations from nine-elevenths to eight-elevenths of his week so he could devote a whole day to his private patients. Alex was in the rooms with Bill on this clinic day and took home the typing, which she did while supervising the children's activities. Bill saw many interesting patients in these rooms. He recalls a Lord Gibson, who had a similar engraving on his signet ring to his own, but with 'a little flourish on each side of the pelican to indicate he was a Lord'. One day when Alex was taking down the details of a Mr Cartier, she asked politely, 'Do you have any connection to the jewellery company, Cartier?' The man replied haughtily, 'Madam, I *am* Cartier'.

A fairly common referral to Bill's private rooms was BPPV, the main cause of short episodes of dizziness associated with someone changing the position of their head or body too quickly. In older people the cause is usually idiopathic (unknown), but in younger people it often results from a head trauma. Bill treated one of the older sisters of the Queen Mother for BPPV and also his former dean of the Middlesex Medical School, Sir Brian Windeyer. It was nearly twenty years since Bill had listened to Windeyer's opening address and it was a surreal experience to now be seeing him 'on the other side of the desk' as his doctor.

It also felt strange for Bill when former superiors from his training days became his colleagues. When the elderly Mr Rotter finally retired at Golden Square, Bill was sucessful in securing a locum consultant post there and resigned from his other locum role at University College Hospital. At Golden Square, Bill worked with his former boss Tony Bull, who did 'beautiful noses', and was allocated one of the those 'very handy' car spaces, opposite the 17th-century plague pit. Golden Square was one of the two branches of the Royal National Throat, Nose and Ear Hospital, so Bill also had access to the other branch in Gray's Inn Road, where he had formerly worked for Harry Beagley.

Bill saw patients from the Outpatients Department at Gray's Inn Road and also sat on a research committee, which he says 'doled out' small grants to allow reseachers to pursue their projects. It was through this committee that Bill first met its chairperson, Lady Pauline Ashley, whose husband Jack, Lord Ashley of Stoke, had lost his hearing in a failed ear operation in 1968.[10] Despite his profound deafness, Lord Ashley was a member of the British parliament. He was also one of the most famous deaf people in Britain after lobbying extensively for the rights of people with disabilites, including those affected by the morning sickness drug thalidomide.

Bill was also part of a small research group called 'Project Ear' which aimed to develop their own cochlear implant. Meetings were conducted at the London Otological Centre and led by his former boss Andrew Morrison, who Bill notes was always 'a most forward-thinking man'. Others on the small committee included Ted Evans, from Keele University, and Richard Balfour-Lynn in an executive role. They were one of only a few groups in the UK exploring the use of cochlear implants. Another group comprised Adrian Fourcin and Ellis Douek, with their 'extra-cochlear' device. There was also Graham Fraser and John Graham at University College Hospital, who developed their own single-channel implant after initially using a device developed by Michael Merzenich and Bob Schindler from the University of California in San Francisco.[11]

Bill was able to explore what was happening on the cochlear implant scene in the US during two separate trips he made during 1982. The first was to the west coast, where he mixed his academic interests with pleasure by taking his family on a three-week touring holiday, taking in Universal Studios and the Grand Canyon before finishing up at the home of Irv Arenberg in Denver, Colorado. The Gibson family had flown into Los Angeles and stayed with Derald Brackmann on the outskirts of the city in Pasadena. Bill accompanied Brackmann to the House Ear Institute, where he met about a dozen surgeons including William and Howard House as well as Howard's son John. Both the institute and William House had become famous for their single-channel cochlear implant. Derald Brackmann took Bill and Alex to a fundraiser for the institute where the entertainment was provided by Bob Hope, who told jokes and sang songs with his second wife Dolores.

The reason Bill and Alex returned to the US during the same year was that Bill had received a letter from the Royal Society of Medicine advising him that he had been chosen as the Smith Kline Visiting Professor for 1982. Bill was introduced for the first time as Professor Gibson when he spoke about his electrophysiology work in at least eight cities across the eastern states, including Boston, New York, Oklahoma City and Dallas, Texas. It was in Houston, Texas, that Bill was very pleased to meet Alfred Coats, the director of the Division of Space Life Sciences at the Universities Space Research Association. Coats had developed a method to replicate

Bill's ECochG results in Menière's patients which did not require the doctor to pierce the eardrum and therefore made it more acceptable in the US.[12]

It was not really a surprise when, in the middle of this hectic year of travelling, Bill received a letter from Barry Scrivener enclosing the job advertisement for Sydney University's newly created Chair of Otolaryngology, with a closing date of 31 August 1982. Bill flew to Sydney for a few days to attend the interview and stayed with Bob. Even though he had previously been encouraged by Scrivener to apply for the position, the vice-chancellor at the university, John Ward, told Bill, 'We'll let you know the outcome, but don't get your hopes up as we also have some Australians in the running'.

* * *

As Bill walked along the verdant lawns of Queen Square and gazed up at his red-brick hospital building, with its steep roof and dormer windows, he felt sad to be 'breaking up the team'. This included his operating partner Alan Crockard and also the neurologist Sir Roger Bannister, with whom he had shared an office for the past four years. During this time, Bill co-authored several clinical papers with Bannister on a type of Parkinson's disease called Shy-Drager, where patients experience paralysis of their vocal cords.[13] Bill says that Roger Bannister had remained a keen jogger since cracking the four-minute mile on a cinder track in Oxford in 1954, but his running days had ended abruptly after a serious car accident. Afterwards, dizziness was a problem, and Bill treated his BPPV in their shared office, using the same vigorous head-shaking exercises he had used on Sir Brian Windeyer to dislodge the otolith particles floating in a semi-circular canal of the inner ear.

Bannister took Bill by surprise one day when he strode into their office and demanded, 'Is it true? Have you really accepted a job in

Australia?' Bannister had attended the opening of the Commonwealth Games in Brisbane in October 1982 and met Richard Guy, the dean of the University of Sydney Medical School, who had asked him, 'What's Bill Gibson like?' Bill says that he had been cautious about sharing the news until his appointment was more certain:

> It was a major decision, because Alex and I had kids still in school and both sets of parents alive. We felt terrible because we knew we'd be taking their grandchildren away from them. Initially, the Professorial Chair at the University of Sydney didn't exist. But then when it did, we thought about it for about one month and decided to go for it.

Theories abounded among Bill's associates about why he wanted to leave one of the top ENT consultant positions in London. Some close friends thought he wanted to leave behind sad memories of his younger daughter. Colleagues thought he liked the idea of becoming a professor, but there was only one Chair of Otolaryngology in London at this time and it was occupied by Donald Harrison at the Royal National Throat, Nose and Ear Hospital in Gray's Inn Road. In fact, for many years after his appointment in 1962, Harrison was the only professor of this specialty in Britain.[14] Bill says the real reason was that he was feeling 'stifled' in his current position and was finding it difficult to fit his academic interests around his NHS commitments. An academic appointment in Sydney, with his own research staff, sounded appealing and showed greater promise than remaining in London.

It was a nice surprise when Bill received a telephone call from Professor Graeme Clark of the University of Melbourne, who was in London and asked if they could meet. After Clark had delivered his talk at the Royal Society of Medicine (RSM), Bill remembers going up to the café on the first floor to have lunch together. Clark had a goatee at the time, which gave him something of 'a mad scientist look'. 'Graeme knew I was going to be working in Australia in the equivalent role to him and made a point of arranging to meet me,' says Bill. 'It was probably more of a highlight for me than him.' Since 1970, Clark had occupied the Professorial Chair of Otolaryngology at the University of Melbourne, which coincidentally had been named the William Gibson Chair after a benefactor.

In the design of his cochlear device, Clark had ignored the sceptics who said it was unnecessary and even dangerous to insert multiple electrodes inside the cochlea. The prototype device Clark had already implanted into two men in Melbourne in the late 1970s had twenty-one electrodes, of which ten were activated and eleven were grounded. A commercialised version of this device had twenty-two activated electrodes and was currently undergoing a clinical trial of six patients in Melbourne. Clark's vision for deaf people was for them to hear the complete speech range, rather than just the morse-code-like signals produced by William House's single channel device. That day over lunch at the RSM, Graeme Clark said to Bill, 'I hope you'll work with me on the cochlear implant program in Australia'.

This was an exciting offer as the Project Ear Group in London were still a fair way off finalising the design of their own cochlear device. This unusual device utilised a receiver implanted in the patient's chest with a wire running up under the skin of their neck to five or six electrodes implanted inside the cochlea. Only time would tell if Bill made the right decision to abandon Project Ear in London and adopt the Australian-designed cochlear implant, which Clark rather optimistically referred to as the 'bionic ear'.

Right up until March 1983, letters and faxes flipped backwards and forwards between Bill's home in Muswell Hill and the vice-chancellor's office at the University of Sydney, finalising his work arrangements. Bill had already stressed to John Ward during his interview in Sydney the importance of being able to operate on children at the Royal Alexandra Hospital for Children, known as the Children's Hospital, which was walking distance away from the university and RPA.

Bill would already know several people when he commenced working at RPA in October 1983. These included the neurologists Michael Halmagyi and Jonathan Ell, his former and current colleagues respectively at Queen Square. Bill was very pleased to be contacted by another Australian, Henley Harrison, who was a visiting medical officer at the Children's Hospital. Harrison came to meet Bill and his family at their home in Muswell Hill and afterwards Bill and Henley went for a run together on the expansive parklands of Hampstead Heath.

Most summers the Gibson family liked to take their picnic baskets to Hampstead Heath for a classical music concert in the grounds of the 1760s mansion Kenwood House. The finale of the concert was always Tchaikovsky's *1812 Overture*. Bill recalls that during a well-known crescendo at the end of the overture, which 'signifies Napoleon's retreat from Moscow in 1812', the sound of cannons would explode from the trees surrounding the picnic grounds and lake. The cannon fire and fireworks at the end of the concert were always the highlights of the evening for Laura and Hugh.

Bill recalls that Alex was wonderful about the whole upheaval of moving to Australia and the children also coped very well. Hugh had already asked if he could board during his final year of preparatory school at Mill Hill in northern London. The senior girls' school Laura attended, North London Collegiate School, was also close to where Peter and Elvira Carr lived at Harrow on the Hill, so for the first few months after their parents' departure, Laura and Hugh would stay with their grandparents.

A house is only bricks and mortar, but Bill loved their home at 75 Onslow Gardens. Peter Carr had helped with the renovations and the final result had such a good feeling that Bill had thought he would never leave. From their back gate, the Gibson family had access to Queen's Wood, where the children had enjoyed toboganning down the snowy slope in winter. The family could all remember the night they had watched from their top-floor windows the sad spectacle of Alexandra Palace, with its thousands of glass panes, bursting into flames and lighting up the London skyline. It was difficult when it came time to sell their home; however, Bill was staggered by the £125 000 they were offered.

During his final weeks of living in London, some doubts crept into Bill's mind about moving his family to the other side of the world. He said to Alex, 'Are we making a huge mistake?' .They decided that if for any reason it didn't work out in Australia, they would return to London and he would apply for Don Harrison's professorial role at the Institute of Laryngology at Gray's Inn Road when it became available.

Happy that they had now had a fall-back plan, Bill looked forward to living in the same city and country as his brother again and becoming a professor at Australia's oldest university. He had progressed up each rung of the career ladder quickly and had now managed to do it again: a full professor by the age of only thirty-nine. As they climbed the steps of the British Airways aeroplane bound for Australia, Bill and Alex had at least half their lives still ahead of them. That was more than enough time to make a new life in Australia while maintaining close ties to loved ones in the UK.

The new professor

I am going to make a telephone call to Susan Walters, who has a cochlear implant ... to show you how much she can understand.

Bill Gibson

Bill and Alex Gibson flew into Sydney in October 1983 and found a nation in a euphoric mood after winning the America's Cup yacht race. Replays of the dawn celebrations in Perth showed the recently elected prime minister Bob Hawke wearing a white jacket emblazoned all over with the word 'Australia'. When he stated on national television, 'Any boss who sacks anyone today for not turning up at work is a bum', Hawke certainly made a stark contrast for the new arrivals to Britain's 'Iron Lady', Margaret Thatcher.

It had been eleven years since Bill and Bob had shared the camaraderie of both living in London and they had hardly met up during that time. Bill enjoyed the couple of months that he and Alex stayed with Bob and Jan in the north shore suburb of St Ives while he settled into his role as the inaugural Professor of Otolaryngology at the University of Sydney. Bill and his brother still looked incredibly alike at thirty-nine, and he comments that one weekend when he picked up his seven-year-old niece Becky from a birthday party, 'nobody batted an eyelid that I wasn't her actual father'.

During these first months, Bill received several well-meaning invitations from members of the Otolaryngology Association of Australia (OLSA). The first was from the president, Gerald McCafferty, who treated him to lunch at one of Sydney's finest harbourside seafood restaurants, which overlooks Luna Park. Afterwards, as Bill lay on the sofa at Bob's house, feeling green from something he had eaten, his other niece, nine-year-old Jenny, 'entertained' him with her flute practice. Bill also remembers some nice older members of OLSA organising a twilight barbecue with partners one Sunday evening on the deck of Frank Lang's home in Hornsby, where the mosquitoes seemed to prefer the 'sweet blood' of the English guests to that of their Australian hosts.

No one could have extended a warmer welcome or been a closer ally to Bill than Barry Scrivener, then in his mid-fifties. Scrivener hoped his younger colleague would carve out new directions for their specialty as the new head of the ENT Department at RPA.

Bill shared surgical lists with Scrivener in the operating theatres on level six of the hospital's Victorian pavilion building and saw patients in the ENT specialty ward on level eight. Also on this level was the temporal bone laboratory, which Bill notes was 'just pottering along' at this stage. This was where his laboratory technician, Cathy Ball, prepared ear bones which donors had bequeathed to his 'Ear Bank'. After they had been soaked in alcohol for several months, Bill used these bones for reconstructive surgery on patients whose middle ears had been destroyed by disease and children with congenital deformities.

The tiled entrance vestibule of RPA is lined with the marble busts of past medical men and the walls are inset with panels of stained glass depicting Queen Victoria and the coat of arms of her second son, Prince Alfred, after whom the hospital was named. From the foyer, Bill only needed to walk along the hospital's circular driveway and then cross Missenden Road to reach the Outpatients Department in Brown Street.

This is where Bill co-headed a unit with Michael Halmagyi which they renamed 'Hearing and Balance' to better reflect its research and clinical activities. Taking up a lot of space in the unit was Halmagyi's 'ocular tilt centrifuge', which Bill recalls was 'rather fun and spun people around like a fairground ride'. This machine would allow them to continue the research on balance they had begun while working together at Queen Square. Bill managed to requisition a few rooms in this unit for his clinical research fellow, Christopher Game, while other rooms were occupied by the three hospital audiologists he would also be supervising.

Bill was pleased that he had been successful in securing the role of honorary consultant surgeon at the Children's Hospital in Camperdown, because this gave him access to a second hospital with facilities for performing hearing assessments and operations on children. The Children's Hospital was only a ten-minute walk from RPA down Missenden Road and across the other side of busy Parramatta Road. Bill had already met one of the visiting medical officers at the hospital, Henley Harrison, in London and they would now be performing operations on children together.

Bill hoped that this would include cochlear implant operations on children in the not too distant future. Considering that a cochlear implant program using the Australian-designed bionic ear was yet to be established in New South Wales, Bill was uncannily accurate when he predicted that 'by the Year 2000 there should be no such thing as a child born to a life of total deafness'. This quote is taken from an article he wrote for the *University of Sydney News* in December 1983, in which he also predicted that:

Over the next few years I am sure there will be a tremendous surge in the early diagnosis of total deafness, which will be remedied by the 'cochlear implant' or 'bionic ear', creating sufficient sensation of sound for speech to be learnt during the vital speech-formation years of one to six years of age ... Children who today are cut off from normal society because of their inability to speak will be able to attend normal schools and take their place in normal society as adults, experiencing relatively minor disadvantages.[1]

Professor Graeme Clark, from the University of Melbourne, forwarded letters to Bill from people around New South Wales who had made enquiries about having their hearing restored. One letter was from a 58-year-old woman, Shirley Hanke, who had been completely deafened at the age of eleven from an allergic reaction to a school diphtheria immunisation. Bill had to concentrate as he listened to Shirley, whose voice was low and European-sounding despite her being a fifth-generation Australian. Shirley's hearing nerves had received no stimulation for forty-seven years and Bill wondered if they would be able to respond to the bursts of electrical activity produced by the electrodes in a cochlear implant.

The media were very interested in Bill's involvement with the fledgling cochlear implant program in New South Wales. Bob can remember rushing home from work one evening to watch Bill in a television interview explaining how the cochlear implant worked. He points out that 'Graeme Clark's implant was known in Melbourne, but it was something new and controversial in Sydney'.

Bob had forged a successful career in real estate since arriving in Australia in 1972. Even though he worked in the city and Bill worked a few kilometres away at a hospital in Camperdown, people still mistook the brothers for each other. This included the time

Bill was about to insert the needle through a patient's eardrum for a hearing test. The man had an anxious look on his face when he said, 'Oh, I know you. You used to work for Raine & Horne.' Bill replied, without the hint of a smile, 'Oh, I've given that away. It wasn't very interesting selling properties, so I've changed professions since then.'

Bob specialised in commercial real estate, so he couldn't provide much practical advice to his brother and sister-in-law about residential properties, but Jan drove Alex around for open inspections. Bill and Alex decided on an attractive clinker brick home, set well back from Clissold Avenue in the northern suburb of Wahroonga, with schools nearby for Hugh and Laura. Bill thinks that Hugh at twelve was the lucky one as he would be starting high school in the correct year, but he worried that Laura would have a harder time fitting in at fourteen, which is 'not the best age to be put into a new girls' school'.

Just before Christmas, Bill flew back to London to collect the children from Peter and Elvira Carr. His parents drove up from Devon to see them off, and they both looked well as he waved them goodbye. Bill and Alex were excited to be reunited with their children and they spent their first Australian Christmas Day with Bob and Jan at a large family gathering with Jan's sister Annette, who lived in nearby Turramurra. The family were missing their two cats in London, which they had given away to a grateful older couple, so in time they would acquire two Burmese kittens, which they named Bunty and Kunta Kinte, and a black Labrador puppy named Bess.

* * *

Early in 1984, a senior ENT surgeon from Sydney Hospital, Victor Bear, telephoned Bill and said, 'Come with me to see the Top End'. Bill can clearly remember their landing in Darwin, because the Nissen huts alongside the landing strip gave it the feel of an air force base and he had to collect his bag from a tractor on the tarmac. They went to Bathurst Island to make recommendations on treatment options for ear conditions in Aboriginal children, who Bill was shocked to discover many were suffering badly with the chronic ear infection otitis media. This disease was present in about 80 per cent of Indigenous children living in remote communities and caused either temporary or permanent hearing loss.[2]

The red-earthed wilderness Bill witnessed in the Top End, and also on a train trip he made with Alex on the *Indian Pacific* across the parched interior to attend an OLSA conference in Perth, revealed the real Australia. However, there was something quintessentially English about the University of Sydney, where Bill worked a few days each week. The campus has many Gothic-inspired sandstone buildings, including the Oxford-style residential colleges around the perimeter and the Great Hall, modelled on Westminster Hall in London. Bill's office was on the third level of the much plainer Blackburn Building. He didn't like to have a large desk between himself and his patients, but the U-shaped piece of furniture dominating his office was clearly a permanent fixture. Lilia Facchetti-Smith remembers the big desk and the high ceilings of his office from her first appointment for progressive hearing loss, when she found Bill to be such a caring medical practitioner that she has consulted him ever since.

One day Bill's secretary Joan Lehane showed into his office a young doctor, Mike Hirshorn, from the Nucleus Group, best known for their pacemakers. The group's chairman, Paul Trainor, had teamed up with Graeme Clark to commercialise his implant. The results of the first clinical trial of the Nucleus device in Melbourne were variable in the degree of benefit derived by the six recipients[3] but considered sufficiently positive to launch further clinical trials. Hirshorn saved the best part of his visit till last, when he stated, 'I would like to offer you two cochlear implants worth $10000 each'.[4]

Hirshorn placed on Bill's huge desk a round, silicone-coated receiver which was roughly the size of a twenty-cent piece. It had a tadpole-like tail, into which the engineers at the Cochlear division of Nucleus had welded twenty-two electrodes. Mike Hirshorn gave Bill a video demonstrating how the Melbourne surgeon Brian Pyman drilled a shallow bed in the skull to hold the receiver-stimulator package and also how he inserted the 19-millimetre-long tail of electrodes through an opening, called the 'round window', into the cochlea.

At the next ENT departmental meeting at RPA, when Bill sought permission to surgically implant the Nucleus device, some-one said, 'Do you think that's wise? We've been told it's a disaster.' Barry Scrivener, or 'Scrivy' as Bill called him, proved helpful in not only pushing the hospital to go ahead, but in overcoming a second hurdle with a group of self-appointed leaders of the ENT profession who called themselves the Toynbee Club.

The annual black-tie meetings of the Toynbee Club alternated between the Australian Club in Sydney and the equally up-market Melbourne Club in Victoria. After dinner, when the committee asked Bill to outline his intentions as the first Professor of Otolaryngology in Sydney, he mentioned that he was about to start using the Australian-designed bionic ear. There was mumbling around the table and then someone asked, 'What are you doing that for?' Bill was not aware that Graeme Clark was unpopular with some members of the club.[5] The committee were very pro William House and thought Bill should go with his American implant – a single-channel device with only one electrode inside the cochlea.

Bill was distressed by their reaction, but on their way home from the meeting Scrivener said to him. 'Go ahead. Let's just do it!' Now they needed to find two suitable candidates, who Bill thought should be young, still have good speech and be completely deafened in both ears. He knew that choosing the wrong recipient and experiencing a failure at this early stage could mean the end of his dreams for a cochlear implant program in New South Wales.

Bill was with a group of medical students the day 22-year-old Susan Walters arrived at the university with her parents for their appointment. Graham and Margaret Walters told Bill that Sue's world had been turned upside-down four months before by a severe bout of meningococcal meningitis – an infection of the fluid and membranes around the brain. During the seven weeks Sue spent in two different hospitals, her eyesight returned and she was looking forward to hearing again but it never happened. She likened the experience to the 'Cone of Silence' from the television series *Get Smart* being lowered around her and jammed shut so she couldn't even hear her own voice.[6]

Bill used the same ECochG test that he had used extensively in the UK to confirm that Sue was completely deaf. He then asked the Oxford-educated audiologist Denyse Rockey to show Sue the unattractive accessories she would soon need to wear. These included a metal headset with a wire running down to a heavy box, which was the size of a Sony Walkman, she would wear on her belt.

Barry Scrivener found the second recipient: 21-year-old Cathy Simon, who had suffered from poor hearing for most of her life, but about eighteen months before had lost the remainder of her hearing overnight. Cathy told her two surgeons that she felt like she had 'won a million lotteries all at once' when they chose her for the second of two historic operations, lasting five hours each, which took place on Wednesday 15 August 1984.[7] Bill recalls there being about five nurses in the RPA operating theatre that day, but it was Denise Lithgow who passed him the surgical instruments.

A day or two later, Bill saw a headline on the front page of an English newspaper which mentioned a cochlear implant operation and thought to himself, 'How do they know about my operation on Sue?' It was the first implant operation performed by his former colleagues from 'Project Ear', Andrew Morrison and Ted Evans, on a young woman named Jessica Reece. It had taken place on the same day as Bill's first two operations, but unfortunately a wire running underneath Jessica's skin snapped, causing the implant to fail. Until the late 1980s attitudes in the UK were quite conservative, with few people receiving cochlear implants, except in the context of research.[8]

The switch-on is the moment of truth for any cochlear implant recipient. Sue's audiologist, Charles Pauka, established threshold and comfort levels for each of the electrodes in her cochlear implant and then loaded her program, or 'MAP', into her speech processor. Bill recalls a tense few minutes after the system went live before Sue heard her first words and said that she had 'started to feel connected to humanity again'.

Sue was fortunate to have a good memory of what speech sounded like, but she would still need weekly rehabilitation with Charles Pauka. Initially this involved 'closed set' discrimination tests, including sets of everyday words and sentences, where she had a chance of choosing the correct word. It was important not to discourage Sue by progressing too quickly to 'open set' discrimination, where she would be given no contextual clues of what the words would be.

Not long after her switch-on, Sue recalls Bill, or 'Prof' as she calls him, returning to England. This visit had been sparked by a worrying call from his father, during which Bill gathered that his mother was on the way out. 'Dad was a very good general practitioner but he seemed to be in denial about the seriousness of mum's amyloidosis,' says Bill, who worried that the deposits of abnormal protein in his mother's gut would make it difficult for her to absorb food. He suggested to Bob that they fly to England immediately to see their mother, who died within weeks of their visit.

After Bill's return, Cathy Simon shared with him her idea for a self-help group where people with cochlear implants could support each other, like she and Sue were doing. In a photo taken of the pair to accompany their stories in the women's magazine *New Idea*[9] Sue and Cathy were so similar in age, height, slim build and raven hair colour, they could easily have been mistaken for sisters.

After the first meeting of the group on on 1 December 1984, held at the Adult Deaf Society in Stanmore, Bill two-finger-typed the group's first newsletter using his new Apple IIe computer. He wrote that some cricket-like insects were making a racket outside the window of his Wahroonga home so he thought that CICADA might be a good name for the club. Bill proposed that this acronym stand for 'Cochlear Implant Club and Deafness Association', but the word 'deaf' was viewed by some as 'politically incorrect'. Bill replaced 'Deaf' with 'ADvisory', which he thinks was 'bending the rules' but better reflected the club's role of educating prospective recipients about what it is like to have a cochlear implant, by people who actually use one.[10]

* * *

As part of her pre-implant assessment, Shirley Hanke was the first person to be tested using the new 'Wavetek Signal Generator' machine. She had to lie on a narrow examination couch, next to a bank of equipment which included a computer and an amplifier to convert the voltage generated by the Wavetek into current. While Shirley wore what she described as 'Tarzan grips' on her ears, Bill asked his clinical research fellow, Christopher Game, to send minute electric currents through a fine needle inserted through her ear drum. She had to indicate by saying the word 'louder' if her 'experience of sound' increased as Game increased the current. This not only gave Shirley a confidence boost, after so many years of deathly silence, but indicated to Bill that her hearing nerves could convey messages to her brain.

On the day of Shirley's hospital admission, Bill had the unenviable task of telling her husband that the University of Sydney would not agree to supplying the Nucleus device without first receiving payment of $9880.[11] Paul Hanke then had to rush home to Wahroonga to collect his cheque book. A week later, when Shirley and Paul returned to RPA so Bill could remove her twenty-four staples, he suggested they visit a World War II veteran, Lionel 'Mick' Barrie, whose operation was the next day. Mick nearly 'chickened out' after seeing Shirley's huge C-shaped wound and how unsteady she still was on her feet.

Shirley considered that she had a better memory of music than speech, so after her switch-on Charles Pauka took her into a sound-proof room and played her the classical cantata *Carmina Burana*. After months of anticipating what it would be like to hear again, Shirley allowed herself to 'have a little cry'. Her cochlear implant would assist Shirley with her lip-reading and she also benefited in other ways. After regular sessions with Charles and the speech pathologists at RPA, Shirley's voice had a slightly higher pitch, with better volume control, and she knew which words to emphasise. She felt confident to use her 'new voice' the night she and Bill gave a talk entitled 'The bionic ear' at the weekly dinner meeting of the Rotary Club of Turramurra.

The Gibson family lived in the same suburb as the Hankes and when Bill's father came to Australia for a holiday, he was impressed by how Shirley could imitate the calls of the native currawongs, kookaburras and lorrikeets she fed from her back verandah.

Paul Hanke kept a diary of Shirley's appointments and noted that 26 March 1985 was a tiring, emotional day for the implant team in their little corner of the Brown Street Outpatients Department. By the time Shirley and Mick arrived in the afternoon for their mapping session, Bill had already observed the switch-on of a 26-year-old Wollongong woman, Gail Hansen, with the 'prying television camera from the *Terry Willesee Tonight* program' monitoring every stage of the delicate proceedings.[12]

Sue Walters' switch-on had also been filmed, as had her surgery. Now, six months later, for the final segment of her video Bill asked RPA's Audiovisual Department to film a split-screen conversation. Using the clipped enunciation of a BBC announcer, Bill said in the video, 'I am going to make a telephone call to Susan Walters, who has a cochlear implant. The idea is to show you how much she can understand.' There was a short interlude of *Star Wars*-like music before the camera panned to Sue, who was seated in a different theatrical set. After a slightly stilted beginning, during which Sue repeated Bill's questions, she hit her stride:

> Bill: I went to Melbourne.
> Sue: Oh, you went to Melbourne.
> Bill: It rained.
> Sue: It rained. It always rains in Melbourne, doesn't it? Did you have a good time down there?
> Bill: It was good, but for three days it rained.
> Sue: Did you take your family?
> Bill: My son and my daughter. We stayed on a farm.
> Sue: You stayed on a farm.
> Bill: My son shot rabbits.
> Sue: How many did he get?
> Bill: Three, but one had myxo [myxomatosis virus].
> Sue: Oh! So you couldn't eat it?
> Bill: We ate two. Will you be going to the meeting?
> Sue: Is it on Friday?
> Bill: That's it. 6 o'clock.
> Sue: Ok, then. Thanks for ringing.
> Bill: Bye.
> Sue: Bye.

The screen returned full frame to Bill, who stood up, smiled broadly and exclaimed in an excited tone to the cameraman, 'That was perfection. That was very, *very* good.'[13] He marvelled at the fact that Sue's brain had been able to take a set of basic electronic signals and turn them into a complex message – like mentally joining the dots in a puzzle. Bill believes this filmed telephone conversation to be the first demonstration anywhere in the world that a cochlear implant could deliver enough information for the recipient to hear speech without any contextual clues. In other words, true 'open set' word discrimination.

'You can't lip-read the telephone,' says Bill, who took the video to show the dozen or so senior ENT specialists at the next meeting of the Toynbee Club. After the lights went back up, there was a frosty, embarrassed silence with not a single question asked. The chairman said, 'I think we'll move on to the next item'. Bill also showed the video at international conferences, which resulted in American colleagues speaking with Sue on the phone themselves and being able to substantiate Bill's claims.

All new clinical drugs and devices need to be tested and approved by bodies such as the FDA in America and the Therapeutic Goods Administration (TGA) in Australia. Bill's early patients were part of the submission Nucleus made to the FDA and in October 1985 they became the first company to gain approval for a multi-channel device from a health regulatory body.[14] This approval meant not only acceptance in America, but worldwide confidence in the Nucleus device. During the next decade Nucleus, known today as Cochlear, would capture 85 per cent of the world market for cochlear devices. The company has maintained this market dominance until the present day.

Regulatory approval and manufacturing in the Sydney suburb of Lane Cove West were two big ticks for Nucleus, but the main worry for Bill was the $12000 price tag of their device, which he knew people on an ordinary wage couldn't afford. One person who fell into this category was a thirty-year-old Danish man, Torben Albaek, who had emigrated to Australia from Copenhagen when he was six years old. Torben believes he was deafened by meningitis, contracted from a public swimming pool in Sydney's western suburbs when he was fifteen years old.

Torben's cochlear implant might never have become a reality if his family, friends and work colleagues at Telecom Australia (now Telstra) hadn't contributed to the cost of the device. His colleagues organised a raffle and spread the word about his implant in the Telecom newsletter. Bill remembers Torben telling him how pleased he was after receiving the implant to be able to hear the roar of his motorbike, whereas previously he had only been able to feel the vibrations of the machine he used to turn up at CICADA events.

In July 1985, CICADA held their first picnic at Lane Cove River Park. It was attended by cochlear implant recipients along with staff from Nucleus and the two Sydney hospitals with cochlear implant programs: RPA and St Vincent's Hospital. The picnic kicked off with a fun run and Bill was the first to cross the tape, although it was rumoured that some competitors had slowed down for the last hundred metres. 'They were nice and let me win,' says Bill, who received one of Sue Walters' home-made Olympic biscuit medallions. After the barbecue lunch there was a tug of war and a messy game called the raw egg throw, which Sue recalls being Bill's 'big thing', because he had done it before in England. 'Prof is such a fun guy. You don't expect your surgeon to get involved, but he threw himself into all the activities.'

* * *

It took a series of referrals before a trim fifty-year-old businessman named Alan Jones found himself in Bill's office at the University of

Sydney. Alan could no longer derive any benefit from the hearing aids he had worn since the age of twenty-one, and wondered if he'd need to retire early. 'The good professor turned out to be a virtual dynamo, whose enthusiasm was contagious and left me in no doubt that the cochlear implant was the only option for my failing hearing.'[15]

The afternoon before his operation, Alan felt apprehensive about a tiny box of electronics being implanted into his skull, so Bill's secretary rang Sue Walters to see if she could visit a patient at RPA. Alan would later describe the young woman who arrived at his room that day as 'an angel in disguise'.

On the day of his switch-on Alan was disappointed to find that not only did voices sound like 'Donald Duck talking under water', but he could feel his facial nerves twitching. By a process of elimination, Charles Pauka worked out that by deactivating eight of the twenty-two electrodes in Alan's implant, he could prevent the spread of electric current to his facial nerve. Fortunately, Alan was able to do without these eight electrodes, which were mainly located in the high-frequency region of his cochlea.

Alan had a regular appointment with Pauka for his rehabilitation every Friday afternoon at 3 pm and after many months of persistent work could speak on the telephone. It wasn't only Sue Walters and Alan Jones who had by now achieved 'open set' speech recognition – Bill says that Cathy Simon, who was doing a teaching diploma in Brisbane, took directions on the phone from Alex about how to get to the CICADA Christmas party.

Bill and Alex offered their back garden for the party in December 1985, with seating for sixty guests, including patients and professionals, around the family swimming pool. They only had a shoestring budget, so attendees volunteered to collect tables from a nearby private boys' school, cutlery from a local restaurant and fresh produce from the markets.

By 1986, Bill was performing eighteen operations per year using transplants of eardrums and ear bones from human donors, but donations were only just keeping up with demand.[16] The death knell to his Ear Bank was not insufficient donations, but rather HIV/ AIDS. Bill felt confident that the bone transplants (homographs) Cathy Ball helped him to prepare were safe, but from now on his upgraded temporal bone laboratory, with five operating micro- scopes, would mainly be used for research and educational purposes.

The Postgraduate Medicine Department of the University of Sydney had previously offered courses on an *ad hoc* basis, but Bill turned them into events that were both regular and enjoyable. During the first ENT update for general practitioners, he asked participants to choose a humorous pseudonym for the quiz.[17] He awarded a bottle of 'sinus washings' as the prize, which sounds awful but was really a bottle of whisky. The same year Bill offered a three- day course for ENT surgeons and invited his American colleague, Irv Arenberg, to be the first of his overseas presenters.[18] A supply of temporal bones was required for the later of these courses, so Bill made a Mark Antony–style appeal for bequests: 'Friends, Australians, cochlear implantees, give me your ears!'

The publicity surrounding the early adult cochlear implant recipients had resulted in many speaking engagements for Bill. This included a talk on the other side of the university campus at the Shepherd Centre, founded by Bruce Shepherd and his wife Annette in 1970 so preschoolers could be taught speech and lip-reading. After his talk, Bill recalls one of the mothers, Glenda Carter, telling him about her son David, who had Mondini syndrome – a congenital malformation resulting in an incomplete number of turns in the cochlea. It pained Bill to tell Glenda that the bionic ear probably wouldn't work in her son's case.

It was not known exactly which children could benefit from the latest technology in hearing aids, tactile devices and cochlear implants, so during a meeting at the Children's Hospital, a decision was made to form the 'Profound Deafness Study Group'. The aim of the group was to foster collaboration between the various hearing professionals working with deaf children, including ENT specialists, audiologists, speech therapists, teachers of the deaf and also a representative from the NSW Department of Education. By rights, this should have been just the kind of group to support Bill in his quest to establish a children's cochlear implant program in New South Wales. He never expected them to be his biggest obstacle.

CHAPTER 9

Children making headlines

At first [Holly] will recognise her own footsteps, the rain and so on. It will be a few more weeks before she recognises words.

Bill Gibson[1]

At the second annual CICADA picnic, the smell of Alex Gibson's tandoori chicken sizzling on the barbecue hotplate mingled with the aromas of the marinated steak prepared by Charles Pauka. The scales had tipped since the previous year, with patients and their families now outnumbering professional staff. Bill told the attendees the good news that from 5 March 1986 most healthcare funds had started reimbursing the cost of the cochlear implant. He said that thanks were due to Shirley Hanke for her letter-writing campaign, directed at politicians including Prime Minister Bob Hawke. Bill also thanked Mick Barrie for making representations to the Department of Veterans' Affairs, which had decided to reimburse their veterans.

After lunch, the winners of the raw egg throw were Hugh Gibson, now fifteen, and sixteen-year-old David, the youngest patient Bill had operated on to implant a Nucleus device. David was also Bill's first implant recipient who couldn't speak, but communicated effectively using 'cued speech',[2] which involves a combination of lip gestures and positioning of the hands in certain shapes near the person's mouth.[3] David had become used to his own means of communication since being deafened at the age of two and now had the arduous task of learning a new language, which Bill thought was akin 'to an English-speaking hearing person learning Russian'.[4] Bill had also performed a cochlear implant operation on a sixteen-year-old girl named Wendy. Although it was hoped that David and Wendy would pave the way for other teenagers to have their hearing restored, Bill thinks they would have both done a lot better if he had operated on them when they were younger.

Bill had already received enquiries about cochlear implants from the parents of younger children, including Lea and Tony Formosa, whose six-year-old daughter Felicity and three-year-old son Joseph were not only deaf, but had also been diagnosed with Usher Syndrome, which can lead to total blindness. The family lived in Oakdale, 80 kilometres south-west of Sydney, and had suffered a string of tragedies, including a house fire.[5] Emmanuel Margolin, a wealthy property developer who had rezoned large tracts of land in this area, offered to host a fundraiser at his home, Notre Dame, to help raise money for the medical expenses of the Formosa children.

Following the dancing horse show in the arena of the 100-acre Notre Dame estate, Bill gave a speech thanking the guests for buying tickets to the event, which had been catered for and organised by the ladies of the Quota Club of Camden. The Gibson family was given a tour of the owner's private zoo by his notorious minder, Tim Bristow. Afterwards Margolin invited Bill, Alex and Hugh for afternoon tea in his mansion, which had a helipad on the roof.

Margolin told them, 'I'd love to have you stay for dinner, but Neville Wran [then Premier of New South Wales] is coming over later on.'

Bill now had the funds to contribute towards the costs of the cochlear devices for the Formosa children, but he was unsuccessful in gaining approval from the Medical Ethics Board for their operations. Bill had also asked the members of the Profound Deafness Study Group (PDSG) about cochlear implants for Felicity and Joseph, and was told, 'They need to learn to Sign first, so they can communicate'. The group suggested that the money raised by the Quota Club be used to provide Sign Language lessons and speech therapy for the Formosa siblings.

Whenever discussion at the PDSG's monthly meetings turned to Bill's plans for a children's cochlear implant program, he noticed that they tried to dissuade him from proceeding. It would never have occurred to Bill that audiologists and teachers of the deaf could be so averse to the idea of restoring a child's hearing. Bill recalls there being a universal feeling in the 1980s that children with a profound hearing loss should be taught 'total communication'. This involved learning Sign Language and using high-powered hearing aids to amplify the parts of the speech range the child could still hear.

'The deaf child hears the vowel sounds but not the consonants,' says Bill. 'If someone says, "She goes shopping", the child hears, "He go hoppin" and speaks with these sounds.'[6] He says children taught in this way developed such poor speech they could not be understood and, not surprisingly, the Deaf community were unhappy about these attempts to make them speak.

* * *

In October 1986, after attending an ENT conference in Germany, Bill extended his trip to England to visit his father in Dawlish. He discovered that his father had transformed Whickham Cottage into a shrine to his mother. Embedded in the lintel above the front door was a plaque bearing her initials, 'JCG', and John had also propped up the little photo of Jane he had taken with him to the war in front of a vase of dried cornflowers, their special 'remembrance flower'.

Bill told his father how much he, Bob and their respective families had enjoyed his visit to Australia the previous year and asked him, 'When are you coming back to see us, Dad?' John, a tall man, replied, 'Oh, it's a long way and the seats kill me'. Bill said, 'Well, why don't you come business class?' Then John countered with 'Oh, I'm not spending my money on business class. The only thing they give you in business class are china plates.' After a few of these circular discussions, Bill came to the conclusion that his father was happier at home with his memories.

Only a month after his return from England, Bill flew to Auckland for the first cochlear implant operation in New Zealand, on 5 December 1986. Bill provided guidance and moral support to the two ENT surgeons, Bill Baber and Ron Goodey, who operated on an Auckland woman, Florence Woodward. Quite by serendipity, Sue Walters was holidaying in Auckland the same week as this historic operation and happily agreed to Bill's request to visit the first New Zealand recipient. Over the next six months there was a flurry of phone calls across the Tasman Sea between members of the two implant teams. Florence Woodward also sent a letter to be printed in the next CICADA newsletter saying how delighted she was 'to meet a fellow implantee'.

With his heavy travel and professorial responsibilities, Bill sometimes arrived late to CICADA meetings, which were held at the city offices of Better Hearing Australia. The committee members decided it would be more relaxing to hold their meetings in private homes. Sue Walters particularly enjoyed the meetings held at the Gibsons' home, because they sat around an antique dining table for the supper Alex provided and they felt like a family. This sentiment is echoed by many of the early recipients, including Alan Jones. Alan and his wife Robyn were now part of a group of volunteers who met with every prospective implant recipient and their family to answer their questions. They knew from personal experience that 'deafness is a shared disability' which also affects loved ones.

Sonny Bennett thinks of Bill as 'a saint' for restoring his hearing. Sonny lost his hearing and balance as a result of being bitten by mosquitoes carrying a virulent strain of the Ross River virus while on a police diving operation in Brewarrina, a country town in the north-west of New South Wales. He had previously won gold medals at Police Olympics, but this extremely tall, athletic man had been forced to retire from the NSW police force on medical grounds at the age of fifty-three. Sonny initially received the House 3M single-channel implant, but it failed after only thirteen months. Sonny thinks that St Vincent's Hospital subsequently stopped offering the House implant, which he says gave him 'noise', whereas the Nucleus device that Bill implanted gave him 'speech'.

Sonny looks about a head taller than anyone else in a photo taken at the second CICADA Christmas party in December 1986, with most of the first group of twenty adult Nucelus implant recipients present. The party was once again held in the back garden of the Gibson family home. Bill had accepted the offer of a Salvation Army brass band to play Christmas carols, but when he saw the cochlear implant recipients hastily removing their speech processors, it was obvious that they were not enjoying the cacophony of sounds.

This would be the last CICADA gathering with only adults and a few teenage recipients because in December 1986 Bill heard the very welcome news that the Cochlear division of Nucleus had been granted approval to commence a clinical trial of their device in the US, Europe and Australia on children from two to eighteen years of age.[7]

* * *

It was one of Bill's colleagues from the Blackburn Building, a pioneering melanoma surgeon named Professor Gerald 'Gerry' Milton, who brought to his attention the plight of a four-year-old girl who had been completely deafened by meningitis. While Holly McDonell was in the recovery phase of her illness, Bill performed ECochG testing under a general anaesthetic at the Children's Hospital. He told her parents to explore all their options and then come back to see him if they needed his help.

Five months later, in April 1987, Holly's mother Viktorija noticed that Holly rarely spoke any more and when she did her speech sounded babbled. Bill and Alex invited the McDonell family to their home for afternoon tea to meet the adult recipient Alan Jones. Unfortunately, there were no children with the Nucleus device in New South Wales they could meet, but Viktorija was impressed by Sue Walters's ability to hold a twenty-minute conversation on the telephone.

The McDonell family also invited Bill to visit them at their home on the western shores of Pittwater, which is only accessible by boat. In the autumn of 1987 Bill towed his boat from Wahroonga to Bobbin Head and then made the forty-minute trip around to Towlers Bay. Viktorija told Bill that Holly no longer chatted to her brother and would hide from the little boy next door, Jolly, because she could not face being unable to communicate with either of them. Holly's father was a professional fisherman on the Hawkesbury River and Bill knew that the $13 000 cost of the Nucleus device was out of the family's reach.

Bill had performed the surgery on twenty-three people to date, but there were a further eighteen on the waiting list for a cochlear implant, who, like the McDonell family, didn't have private health insurance.[8] The RPA appeals committee had paid for some of Bill's cochlear implant patients, and retailers such as Grace Brothers and

Dick Smith had paid for others, but there simply weren't enough kind-hearted people to go around.

One of Bill's neighbours in Wahroonga took him to meet a businessman, Larry Adler, the founder of FAI insurance, in his Macquarie Street office. Adler, a Hungarian immigrant like Charles Pauka, said he was happy to provide the $13 000 for Holly's Nucleus device. His son Rodney, a chief executive of FAI at this time, pledged to support future upgrades of her speech processor.

Everything was now in place for Holly's operation. Bill even had the printouts of her flat ECochG traces to prove to the other members of the PDSG that she really was deaf. The group was already 'livid' with Bill for agreeing to implant a four-year old, but he says, 'There would have been a complete outcry if I had somehow implanted a hearing child'. A senior official from the NSW Department of Education had already rung Bill to tell him that he should not proceed. Then, on the evening before Holly's operation, the same official travelled by boat to Holly's home to beg her parents to reconsider. She told them that Holly should attend the Deaf Unit at Chatswood Public School (PS). What did they want, the official asked them, 'some kind of miracle?'[9]

Bill asked several surgeons to assist him with the operations on Holly McDonell and the children who followed. These included Barry Scrivener and two surgeons who had visiting medical officer status at the Children's Hospital, Henley Harrison and Ted Beckenham. 'Bill wanted us all there for moral support, but he was the one who actually operated on Holly,' said Harrison of the three-and-a-half hour operation Bill performed on 4 June 1987 at no charge to Holly's parents. The operation took place a week and a half before Holly turned five, placing her at the lower end of the allowable age limit to receive a cochlear implant. She would later be acknowledged on a timeline on the Cochlear Australia and New Zealand Ltd website as 'the first paediatric recipient' worldwide of their cochlear devices.[10]

A few weeks after Holly's surgery, Bill operated on Joseph Silipo, a nine-year-old boy who had been deafened by meningitis when he was nearly four and had been relying on lip-reading ever since. Through sheer determination, this remarkable little boy had managed to retain his speech.

For Holly and Joseph's operations, Bill used a new device, the CI22M or 'Mini', which the Cochlear division of Nucleus had released in February 1987. Like its predecessor, it had the diameter of a twenty-cent piece, but it was about 30 per cent slimmer and included a magnet. This internal magnet aligned with a magnetised transmitting coil the child (or adult) wore behind their ear, so it was no longer necessary to wear a wire headband.

Sue Walters attended Holly's switch-on, during which the therapist established the comfort and threshold levels for only a few of the twenty-two electrodes in her implant, so that she didn't experience too many sounds at once. Bill was quoted in a newspaper article as saying, 'At first, she will recognise her own footsteps, the rain and so on. It will be a few more weeks before she recognises words.' The article appeared in the *Sydney Morning Herald* the day after her switch-on under the headline: 'Holly's world full of sound again'.[11] Alongside the article there was a photo of the first and the youngest recipients of the Nucleus device in New South Wales: Sue Walters, who answered the reporters' questions, and shy little Holly, with her pale blonde hair shaved on one side, who sat through the press conference without saying a word.

Holly required daily habilitation sessions with her mother under the guidance of specially trained therapists and teachers of the deaf. Habilitation sessions assist the child to develop, or redevelop, their listening and language skills after a cochlear implant operation. The program, or MAP, in the child's speech processor would also require regular adjustments by an audiologist. This therapy could take from months to years, depending on the child's auditory memory of sound.

During these early days there was only Bill and one therapist, but as more children received a cochlear implant and funding was obtained, more habiliation staff were employed to join the team. There were several people who played an important role in establishing the protocols for the habilitation of post-implant children over the next few years. These include, but are not limited to, the audiologist Catherine Brown, the teacher of the deaf Anne Fulcher, the aural habilitationist Maree Rennie, and the auditory-verbal therapist Rosalie Yaremko.

* * *

Bill sought the advice of Professor Graeme Clark in Melbourne about the type of hearing professionals he should employ. Clark, who was in his mid-fifties at this time, also agreed to Bill's request for him to be the guest of honour at the first formal evening function of CICADA, held on 30 July 1987. Due to the need to minimise background noise for the cochlear implant recipients, Charles Pauka arranged the hire of a private function room for a sit-down dinner at the Kirribilli RSL Club, where he was a member.

In his after-dinner speech, Clark told the story of a holiday to Minnamurra Beach on the south coast of Sydney in 1977 which provided the solution to the dilemma of how to spiral the electrodes into the cochlea. 'I was playing with turban shells, which are a replica of the cochlea,' said Clark. He noticed that the graded stiffness and flexible tip of a blade of grass inserted into the opening of a turban shell allowed it to wrap around the internal spirals nearly all the way to the centre.[12] Clark said that he rushed home afterwards to try it on a human bone and it was a eureka moment when it worked. He then held up a turban shell for the 130-plus attendees to see.

Several children who were potential candidates for a cochlear implant attended Chatswood PS on Sydney's north shore, which had three classes for deaf children. Whereas the majority of deaf programs used Sign Language, the children at Chatswood PS were taught using an auditory-oral approach. Sylvia Romanik headed this progressive unit and was assisted by two teachers, Maggie Loaney and Helen Dawson. Bill thought this school would be a good place to begin the children's post-implant therapy; however, he could see its limitations in the long term as members of his habilitation team only had a very small room and/or corridor in which to conduct the children's switch-ons and therapy.

One of the deaf children participating in the auditory-oral lessons at Chatswood PS was Pia Jeffrey, who has congenital deafness. Both of Pia's parents carried a gene for deafness which had been expressed in both five-year-old Pia and her two-year-old brother Alex, while their older sister, Kitty, has normal hearing. Prue Jeffrey had been excited about the idea of Pia having a cochlear implant since hearing Bill speak at the Shepherd Centre a year or two before. Pia had few spoken words that were intelligible to others and her parents had been told, 'Pia will never learn to hear and talk. She should just accept the handicap and learn to Sign.'

Historically, congenitally deaf children like Pia, who were unable to speak, were described as being 'deaf and dumb'. Bill says that the words 'dumb' or 'dumm' mean 'stupid' in the Teutonic languages and in the past these people were treated as imbeciles and a source of ridicule.[13] It was a French priest, the Abbé Charles-Michel de l'Epee, who devised the first Sign Language and founded the first public school for deaf children in Paris in 1755. It enabled them to communicate and, in doing so, to demonstrate that they had the same level of intelligence as their hearing peers.[14]

'The Abbé broke the chains away from the Deaf,' said Bill, 'giving them self-esteem and allowing them to enjoy a new sense of freedom.' Many, including Graeme Clark, consider the cochlear implant to be the first major advance for totally deaf children since the development of Sign Language two hundred years before.[15]

Bill operated on Pia on 19 August 1987, only three weeks before her sixth birthday. He believes her to be the youngest born-deaf child in the world to receive the Nucleus device. Media reports about the groundbreaking cochlear implant operations he performed on first Holly McDonell and then Pia Jeffrey inflamed the Sydney–Melbourne rivalry that exists in most scientific and cultural pursuits. However, Bill's intention was always to support rather than compete with Professor Clark's cochlear implant program in Melbourne.

Any interstate rivalry was transient and low-key, but it was members of the Deaf community who Bill really upset by operating on a congenitally deaf child. 'Pia was the one who really caused consternation. I received a sack full of mail, condemning me for putting a cochlear implant into a child who was born deaf.'

A Deaf writer, Michael Uniacke, pointed out the distinction between 'born deaf' and 'acquired deafness' in an article he wrote for the *Weekend Australian* the month after Pia's operation.[16] Uniacke stated that a common source of anger among the Deaf community is that the device 'promotes the idea that to be deaf is to be sick'. Uniacke was quoted in the article as saying, 'I'd go crazy if I got part of my hearing back. It would be the equivalent for me of losing a part of my soul.'

An Australian parenting magazine accused Prue Jeffrey and her husband John of being irresponsible parents for making the decision on behalf of their child for her to have a cochlear implant. Prue says that Pia had her bag packed with her favourite book and soft koala several weeks before she was admitted to the Children's Hospital. Bill had given the family a video of an operation and switch-on of the first patient from the Melbourne cochlear implant program, 46-year-old Rod Saunders, but he warned Pia's parents that 'It's a bit too gory for a little girl of five'. During Rod's switch-on, when he can be seen laughing as he hears his first sounds, Prue and John realised that Pia had climbed out of bed and was now pointing animatedly at the screen and then to her own chest.

From a medical point of view, Bill was entering unchartered waters. He says that on the day of Pia's switch-on, 'We were on tenterhooks because we weren't sure if it was going to work'. Pia rested her fingers pensively on her lips as she waited for the first words to come through, which were 'Hello, hello, hello'. Her face suddenly changed. 'Hello', Pia said back. Then she stopped so she could listen to her own voice say once again the word 'Hello'. Holly's responses to sound were quoted as part of the cover story in the Saturday 19 September edition of the *Sydney Morning Herald*, which bore the headline: 'Tears as Pia hears her first voice'.[17] Dominating the front page was a series of five photos leading up to the moment when Pia broke into a smile, with both hands cupped around her face.

Walking past a news stand on the Saturday of the cover story, Bill's son Hugh, who was aged seventeen at the time, noticed a broadsheet in a wire holder with the same photo of Pia, but much larger, under the banner heading 'Pia's first sounds'. He brought it home for Bill, who had it framed.

Pia's teachers had to go back to the beginnings of language development for her habilitation, but in her first session she could discriminate between one-syllable words such as 'cat' and three-syllable words like 'elephant' and 'butterfly'.[18] Pia's mother was present for her habilitation sessions and then worked with her daughter at home for an hour each day. On the day of Pia's sixth birthday party, only a week after her switch-on, it was the sound of tearing paper that caught her attention. Bill and Alex attended the party and Prue was touched by the long birthday banner Bill produced on his home computer and 'daisy wheel printer'.

Bill remembers Prue telling him that Pia was enjoying the sound of the toilet flushing so much she had 'milked the system dry'.

Henley Harrison says that cochlear implants in children were new territory and it took a long time to see the results. 'In the meantime, the naysayers were ready to pounce on anyone with a poor outcome. Bill loves kids and he broke down the barriers to younger children receiving implants and being given hearing and speech,' says Harrison, who considered this to be 'an earth-shattering thing for Bill to have achieved'.

* * *

Bill had been waiting for an opportunity to explain to someone prominent in government the difficulty he was having funding cochlear implants for public patients. That opportunity arose in mid-1987 at the annual RPA medical consultants' dinner. The NSW Health Minister, Peter Anderson, remembers standing up to leave the dinner when the general superintendent of RPA, Diana Horvath, introduced him to 'a quietly spoken professor' named Bill Gibson. Bill asked Anderson if he believed in equitable access to healthcare and when he replied that he did, Bill asked: 'What would you say is the answer to someone who needs a cochlear implant but they don't have private health insurance or a wealthy benefactor to pay for them and there's no government funding. I have twenty such people on my waiting list.'

Not long after the dinner Bill heard the good news that Anderson had delivered on his promise to annually fund ten cochlear implants for adults, equalling a cash injection to his implant program of $150000 per year, indexed for inflation. The day after the announcement, an article was published in the *Sydney Morning Herald* which stated that 42-year-old Carole Cullen from Gorokan on the NSW central coast was currently at the top of the waiting list for a cochlear implant.[19] When Bill operated on Carole at RPA, she became the first publicly funded patient in New South Wales to receive a cochlear implant.

The next child Bill performed cochlear implant surgery on was four-year-old Alison Vary, who had been deafened by Ross River virus – the same infection that had deafened the former policeman Sonny Bennett. In an article that filled the front page of the Lismore *Northern Star* on 6 November 1987, Alison's father said, 'While she was deaf, her little face was drawn and she never smiled … It must have been frightening for her – not knowing what was happening.'[20]

Alison fulfilled all the criteria for a cochlear implant, except living close enough for the post-implant habilitation. The solution Bill proposed was that a speech pathologist from Casino Memorial Hospital be trained in Sydney and then conduct weekly sessions with Alison near her home on the mid-north coast of New South Wales. This was after Alison and her family spent a school term in Sydney so she could receive daily habilitation.

Alison was wearing her speech processor tied to the front of her flouncy dress the day she and her family attended the luncheon at the McDonells' home, which overlooked the blue, protected waters of Towlers Bay. This luncheon, in December 1987, was an opportunity for Bill and members of his children's cochlear implant program to celebrate the significant milestones they had achieved during the previous year, and many prominent doctors and businesspeople were in attendance. They included Professor Gerry Milton, who owned a holiday house next door, and the chairman of the Nucleus group, Paul Trainor, who pushed Alison on a red tricycle up a dirt track through the gum trees towards the house. Many of the adult implantees attended the lunch, including Shirley Hanke. She recalls her husband Paul saying that even when he stood behind Holly to hold the binoculars in front of her eyes, she could still hear him clearly.

Within six weeks of the completion of her switch-on, Holly's speech had returned and she was able to resume many of the play and reading activities that had ceased as a result of her deafness. Viktorija McDonell remembered the question posed to her the night before her daughter's cochlear implant operation by the education official and thought to herself, 'That miracle? I think we got it.'[21]

The guests at the luncheon had arrived by ferry from Church Point or by 'hitching a ride' on the McDonell family's professional fishing trawler. Bill arrived at the McDonell's jetty in his own boat and brought with him his friend Richard Ramsden, who was the first of his former colleagues from the United Kingdom to visit Sydney and lead one of his temporal bone courses for ENT surgeons. During his stay, Ramsden sent a postcard to David Moffat, the third member of 'The London Triumvirate', featuring a photo of a sinewy old bushman in a loin cloth. The message on the reverse of the postcard read, 'Bill has really aged since coming to Australia'.

Bill missed his London friends, but a return to the United Kingdom seemed very unlikely now. Australian citizenship was a requirement of the Rotary exchange program that Laura and Hugh were both keen to undertake during their gap years so the whole Gibson family turned up at the Ku-ring-gai Council chambers to become naturalised Australian citizens. They met the mayor and had their photo taken by Shirley Hanke, who worked at these same chambers. Laura then left for her gap year at a girls' school in Port Elizabeth in South Africa.

Holly McDonell also embarked on her first day of school, but in her case it was in the kindergarten class at Mona Vale Public School on Sydney's northern beaches. Holly would later reflect on the huge decision her parents made on her behalf regarding whether to send her to a special school for the deaf and said, 'Having faith in me, they opted for the local public school.' Her mother Viktorija said, 'Holly [has] no real problems in listening and comprehension in a class of thirty students. My husband and I, as parents of a child with a bionic ear, are very pleased with Holly's progress, which has exceeded our hopes and expectations.'

Viktorija wrote these words as the mother of a child with a cochlear implant in a letter to the editor of the *SHHH* (Self Help for Hard of Hearing People) *News*. Adult implant recipients, including Shirley Hanke, also wrote a letter to this newsletter in response to their February 1988 issue, in which Michael Uniacke had published another article criticising the cochlear implant. Most of the article that appeared in *SHHH News* had been reprinted word-for-word from a previous article by Uniacke in the magazine of the Commission of the Future, *In Future*, under the same headline: 'Of miracles, praise – and anger – The Bionic Ear'.[22]

Over the previous few years, Bill had become accustomed to reading articles criticising the cochlear implant and also his own children's and adults' cochlear implant programs, but he never expected to have accusations made about him by a disgruntled former team member. He was about to experience one of the most stressful periods of his life, when a lesser man might have been tempted to pack his bags and return to England.

CHAPTER 10

Storm clouds

I regret that a cloud covers the EAR
Foundation and until this has been
investigated and cleared, it would be
unfair to the Governor-General of the
Commonwealth of Australia or any of
our supporters to continue with
the dinner.

Bill Gibson

Bill was keen to perform cochlear implant operations on more
children, but having his staff do their switch-ons in a storeroom
at Chatswood PS was clearly not a sustainable solution. He was currently conducting the electrical testing on children at the 2UE Hearing
Assessment Unit, located in Wade House in the grounds of the
Children's Hospital. The hospital's general superintendent, John Yu,
was agreeable to Bill acquiring some space on the level below this
unit as long as he could raise sufficient funds for the renovations.

The cochlear implant surgeon at St Vincent's Hospital, John
Tonkin, introduced Bill to Arthur Yenibis, who owned a clothing

factory near Central railway station. This cigar-smoking Greek businessman offered $50000 towards the refurbishments, so Bill proposed that they name the new centre after him. The hearing professionals in the PDSG thought the centre was suited to the fitting of not only cochlear implants but also hearing aids and tactile devices. They collaborated with Bill on the production of a brochure to attract further donors to the Yenibis Deafness Research Centre.

Funding was difficult to procure for something as new and controversial as the cochlear implant, so Bill will be eternally grateful to Peter Anderson for being the first NSW Minister for Health to provide an annual grant for his adult implant program. Anderson relinquished this role to Peter Collins following the change of government in March 1988, but he was still the natural choice as the guest of honour for the second CICADA sit-down dinner two months later on 25 May.

In a photo from the evening, Sue Walters can be seen wearing a red ribbon and bow on the metal headband which kept the transmitting coil of her speech processor in place. Implantees had various names for this metal headband, ranging from 'Alice band' to 'the birdcage', but if the transmitting coil in this headset was even 5 to 10 millimetres off-centre, the communication link to the internal components of the implant was broken. In 1988, the Cochlear division of Nucleus released its 'magnet option' for people like Sue, who had the original Nucleus 22 device. This option included a titanium-encased magnet with three small legs which allowed surgeons to anchor it in place over the existing implant in an hour-long surgical procedure.

There was usually some trial and error regarding the positioning and strength of the magnet inside the transmitting coil, and adjustments could be made by the clinic staff with a screwdriver. The magnet needs to be in the correct position so that the coil adheres to the back of the person's head, behind their ear. However, if the magnetic force holding the coil in place is too strong, it can cause skin irritation at the point of contact.

Shirley Hanke encountered a different problem. In her case it was static electricity, when, for example, she pulled a synthetic garment over her head without first removing the plastic-covered magnetised coil. One particularly dry, windy day, Shirley entered a carpeted room and static electricity produced an intense burst of electrical stimulus in her speech processor. She felt what she described as 'a kind of explosion' in her head, leaving it sore for weeks afterwards, and Cochlear staff supplied her with a newly programmed speech processor.

Jim Patrick, an engineer who now headed the research team of this division, heard similar reports from other cochlear implant centres overseas and says this led to design changes to the implant and speech processor. Many of Bill's cochlear implant recipients, including Shirley, visited the Nucleus headquarters on a regular basis to be tested and provide feedback on their experiences.

* * *

The first child to have surgery in the second phase of the children's cochlear implant program was three-year-old Alex, the younger brother of Pia Jeffrey. Photos of the siblings hugging each other tightly appeared in newspaper articles at regular intervals. A Deaf activist, Colin Allen, stated in the *Sydney Morning Herald*: 'I am tired of the story of Pia Jeffrey — all the newspapers saying: "The world of sound is opened up". So other parents say, "Gee, I want that for my child".'[1]

It can be difficult for hearing people to understand why some members of the Signing Deaf community were so opposed to cochlear implants. For Bill, it was an incident during a stay with his North American colleague Irv Arenberg that opened his eyes to analogous situations with other disability groups. Bill and Irv collaborated on some of the very early research on the use of ECochG as a monitoring tool during inner ear surgery.[2] They presented their findings at symposiums organised by the Prosper Ménière Society in Colorado and on such occasions Bill would arrange a visit to Arenberg's palatial residence in Greenwood Village, a suburb of Denver.

Unable to sleep one night, Bill switched on the television in Irv's downstairs guest room and came across a program about the 'Little People of America', which discussed attempts to cure dwarfism with hormone treatments and/or surgery. The program highlighted the case of a teenage girl who had endured a series of surgical procedures to lengthen her limbs. When the girl said, 'I can now play netball with my friends', the studio audience chanted, 'Traitor, traitor!' The host of the television program said, 'That's a disgrace … You were born to be a dwarf.' This reminded Bill of comments made by Deaf groups about congenitally deaf children: 'You were born to be Deaf and part of a Signing community.'

The next congenitally deaf child Bill operated on was a toddler named Amelia Hardy, when she was two years and ten months old. Her mother Renee said that Amelia loved running around their farm at Jamberoo on the NSW south coast, but that it was pointless to call out to her, 'Look out for the tractor!' or 'Don't go near that!' Naturally, it was a major breakthrough for her parents the first time Amelia turned around when her name was called. A photo of Amelia holding a Raggedy Ann doll and sitting opposite the adult recipient Alan Jones appeared on the cover of a Cochlear 'Issues and Answers' brochure and was a portent of her future modelling career.

In September 1988, soon after performing Amelia's cochlear implant surgery, Bill operated on an even younger child, Andreas, who was two years and one month old. In a story which featured on the front page of the *Manly Daily*, Andreas's mother said that she had

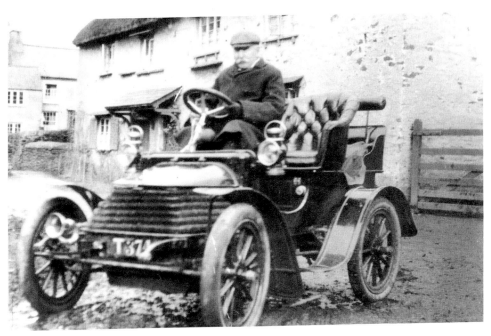

Great-grandfather George Gibson (1844–1931) owned some of the first cars in Devon, including this pre-World War I Wolseley.

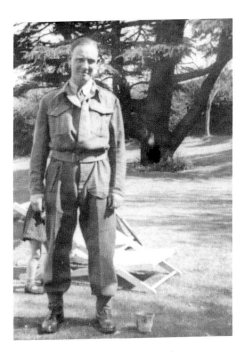

Captain John Gibson, home on leave in Totnes, Devon, in April 1944, in the garden of Lakemead with the cedar tree in the background.

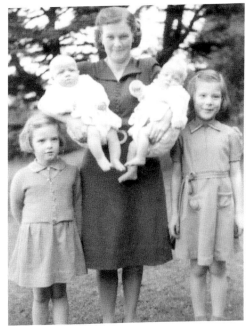

Jane Gibson in October 1944, holding her four-month-old twin sons Bill and Bob, with Kathy (age four), to her left and Eleanor (age seven), to her right.

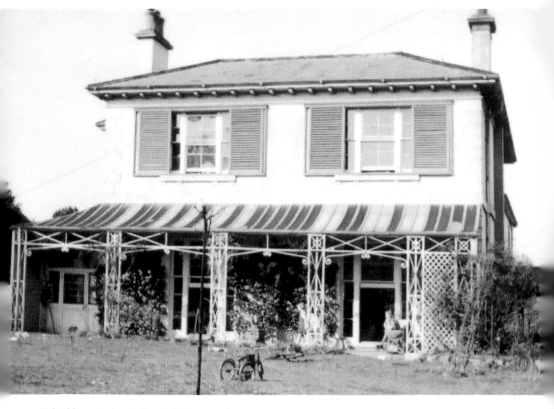

Whickham Lodge in Dawlish, Devon, circa 1947.

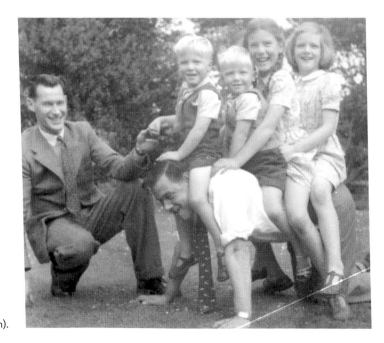

The Gibsons' lodger, Fred Lloyd, and a friend, provide amusements in the garden for Bill and Bob (age four), Eleanor (age eleven) and Kathy (age seven).

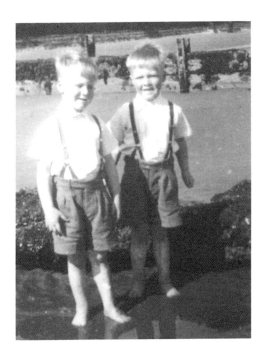

Bill (right) and Bob, aged seven, by the seaside in Dawlish.

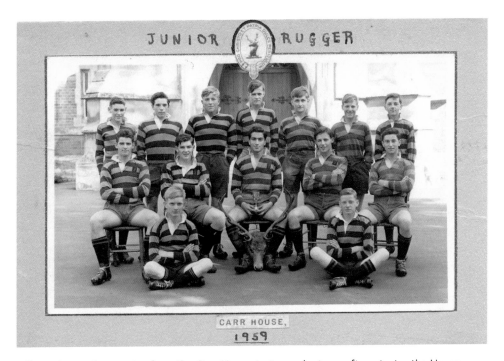

Bill, aged 15, with teamates from the Carr House junior rugby team after winning the House Cup in 1959. Back row: Hardstone, Bush, Turner, Roberts, Dyke, Gibson and Stober. Centre row: Peall, Holmes, Fattal (captain with stag's head), Newson-Smith and Werber. Front row: Coe and Allen.

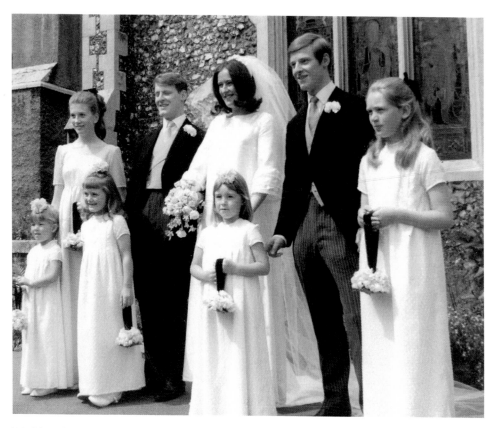

Wedding day at St Mary's Church of England at Harrow on the Hill, 15 June 1968.
Back row: Elspeth Pearson, Bill and Alex Gibson, Bob Gibson and Julie Makey.
Front row: Catherine Marshall, Jocelyn Brown and Sally Marshall.

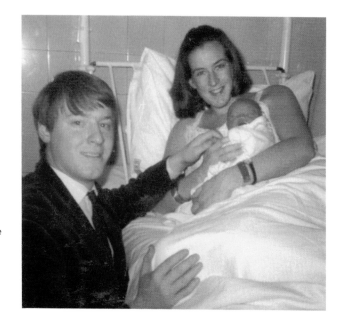

Although not close in distance from Harrow on the Hill, Bill and Alex chose the very familiar Middlesex Hospital for the birth of Laura Louise in December 1969.

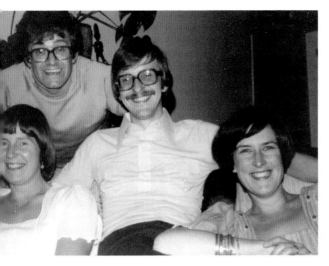
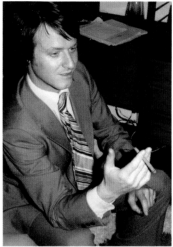

A dinner party to celebrate Bill's appointment as a consultant at Queen Square, 1977. From left: Wendy and Richard Ramsden, David Moffat and Alex Gibson. And Bill, top right, holding a slim cigar and looking suave at the same dinner party.

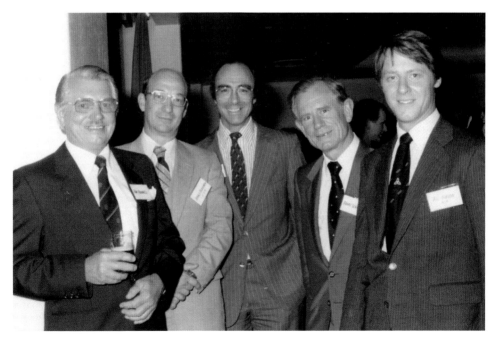

Leaders of a neuro-otology course at the University of Sydney, 1981, including from left: Tom O'Donnell, Derald Brackmann, Paul Fagan, Barry Scrivener and Bill Gibson, who took leave from Queen Square in London to attend.

Alex, Laura (age 15), Hugh (age 13) and Bill in the courtyard of their new home in Sydney, with their Labrador Bess in the foreground, 1984.

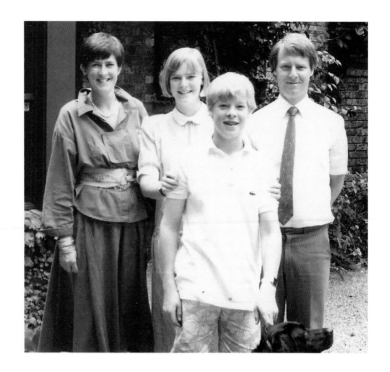

Bill with some recipients of the Nucleus and 3M cochlear devices who attended a Christmas party at his home, 1986. Back row from left: Arthur Haggarty, Kath Westbrook, Tracey McDonald, Cathy Simon, Bill Gibson, Clifford Elliot, Shirley Hanke, Sonny Bennett, Sue Walters, David Suutari and Alan Jones. Front row from left: Kath Mackie, Kazuko Scott, Lynette Moncaster, Joan Shying, Gordon Parish and Valerie Sexton.

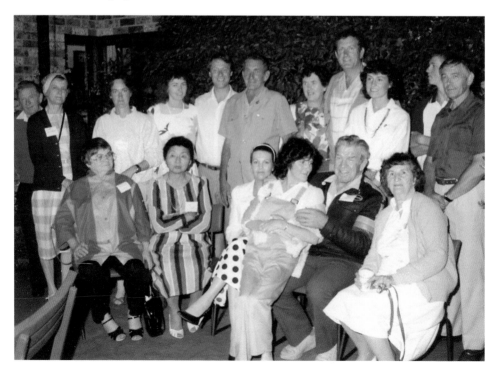

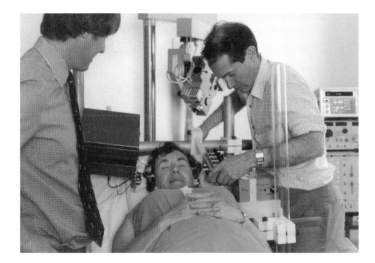

Bill observes Christopher Game using the Wavetek machine to test if Shirley Hanke experiences any 'sensation of sound' after 47 years of silence.

Shirley reveals her huge C-shaped wound, three weeks after cochlear implant surgery at RPA, February 1985.

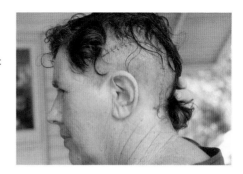

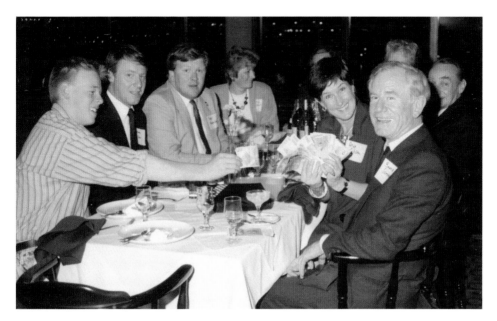

CICADA dinner at the Kirribilli RSL Club, 25 May 1988. From left: Hugh and Bill Gibson, Peter Anderson (former NSW Minister for Health), Robyn Jones, Alex Gibson, Barry Scrivener and Paul Trainor (far right).

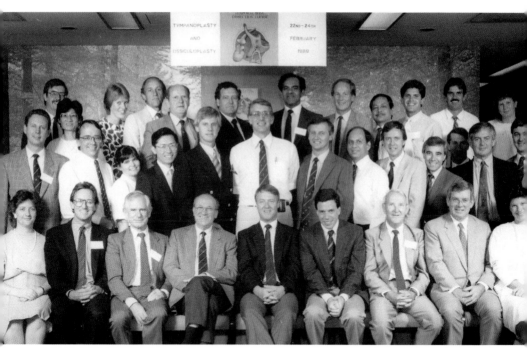

Temporal Bone Dissection Course at Sydney University, 22–24 February 1989. Seated in front row from left: Christine Woods (lab technician), David Pohl, Barry Scrivener, Michel Portmann, Bill Gibson, René Dauman, Jack Lancken, Brian O'Reilly and Denise Lithgow (registered nurse).

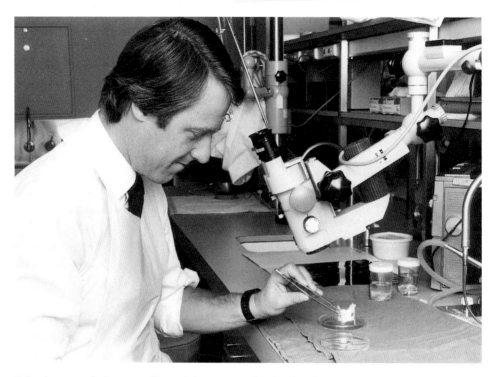

Bill in his upgraded temporal bone laboratory on level eight of RPA, examining a bone donation (homograph).

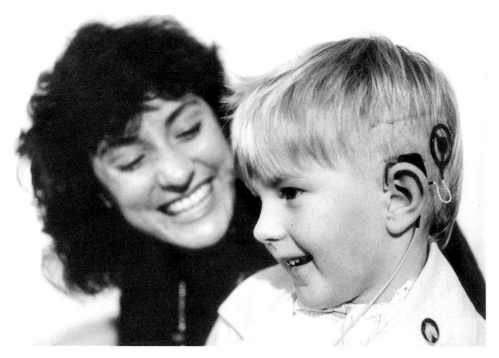

The first and the youngest recipients of the Nucleus device in NSW, Sue Walters and Holly McDonell, at a press conference, 9 July 1987. *Anton Cermak, Fairfax Media*

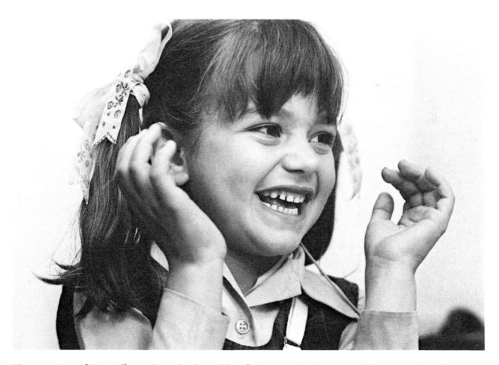

The reaction of Pia Jeffrey when she heard her first sound at six years old appeared on the front page of the *Sydney Morning Herald* on 19 September 1987, under the headline, 'First, waiting for the miracle...Then with the flick of a switch...'. *Rick Stevens, Fairfax Media*

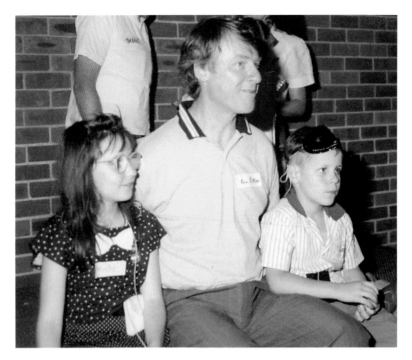

Seated on either side of Bill at the CICADA Christmas party, held at the Villa Maria school hall, are Felicity and Joseph Formosa (aged eight and five respectively), both of whom are deaf and have Usher Syndrome, which can lead to total blindness.

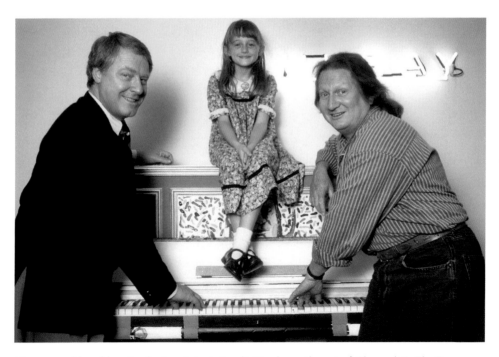

Nine-year-old cochlear implant recipient, Amelia Hardy, on the set of Channel 7's *The Doug Mulray Show*, sits on top of a piano with Bill to her left and Doug Mulray to her right, 1994.

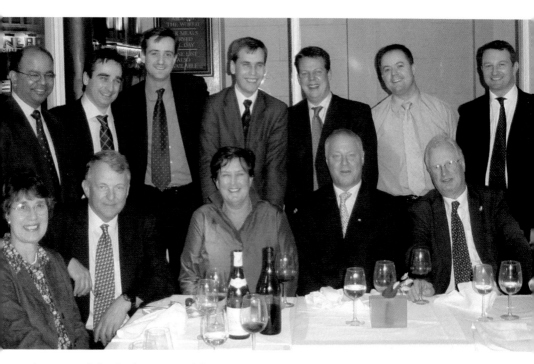

A reunion of the Graham Fraser fellows who came to Australia to be trained by Bill, London, 2003. Back row from left: David Selvadurai, Brendan Conlon, Peter Rea, Tim Mitchell, Peter Valentine, Simon Hargreaves and Nicholas Mansell. Front row from left: Graham Fraser's widow Patricia, Jonathan Hazell (trustee), Alex and Bill Gibson, John Graham (trustee).

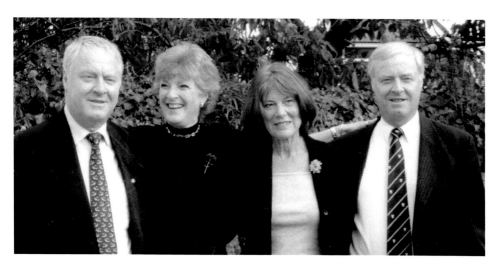

Bill (left) with Kathy, Eleanor and Bob before their father's funeral in October 2001. Bill's sisters both wore a cornflower, which was their parent's special 'remembrance flower'.

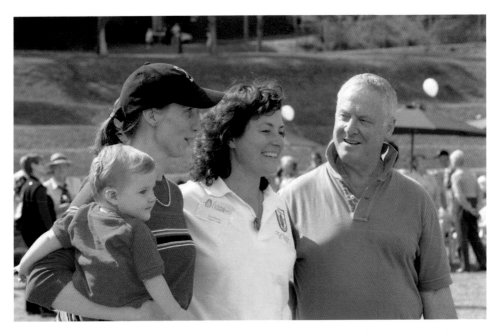

A picnic to celebrate the SCIC's 1000th cochlear implant operation, with marquees on the cricket oval of the Old Gladesville Hospital, 19 September 2004. From left: Cathy Birman, holding 11-month-old Ruby Loosemore in her arms, with Sue Walters and Bill.

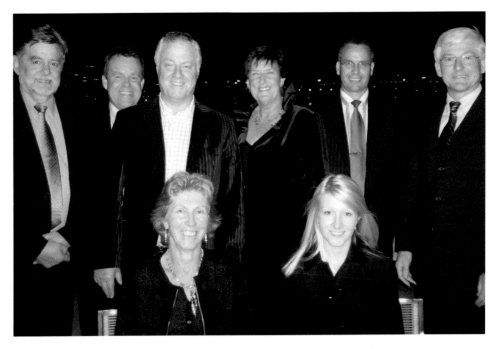

A dinner in 2007 near Sydney Harbour hosted by the executives of Cochlear Limited to celebrate the 20th anniversary of the operation Bill performed on Holly McDonell, who was the first paediatric recipient in the world of the bionic ear in 1987. Back row from left: Jim Patrick, Shaun Hand, Bill and Alex Gibson, Chris Rehn and Chris Roberts (the then CEO of Cochlear). Front row: Viktorija and Holly McDonell.

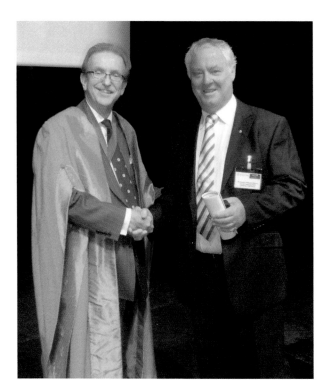

Bill receives a BACO gold medal from David Moffat, the master of the British Academic Conference in Otolaryngology, when it was held in Liverpool, July 2009.

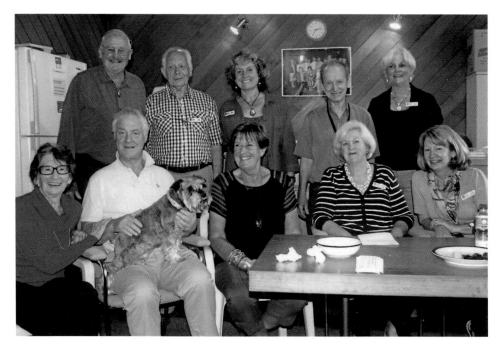

CICADA committee members in their club room at the SCIC, 2010. Back row from left: Peter Keegan, Alan Jones, Sue Walters, Neville Lockhart and Judy Cassell. Front row from left: Roma Wood, Bill with Lilly (the miniature schnauzer), Alex Gibson, Chrissy Boyce and Karen Cooper.

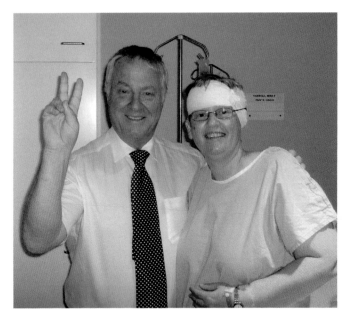

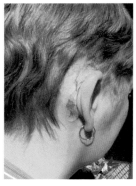

Faye shows the 'small, straight incision' behind her ear, which was developed by Bill to reduce the rate of wound breakdown.

Bill holds up two fingers to indicate a second cochlear implant for Faye Yarroll, who can be seen two hours after her surgery at the Mater Hospital.

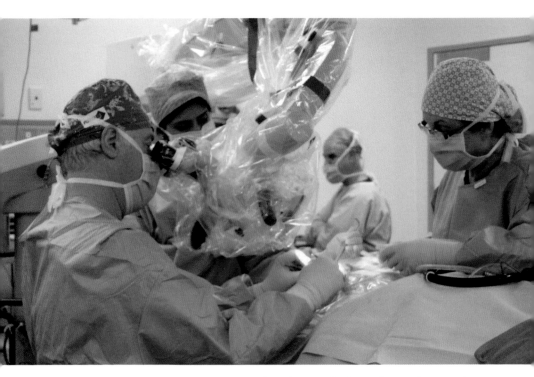

Cochlear implant surgery at the Mater Hospital on the day of a farewell party from the theatre staff to Bill, who is looking down the eyepieces of the operating microscope with Payal Mukherjee, November 2013. To their right is the scrub nurse, Carol Macdonald, and behind them is the bioengineer, Halit Sanli.

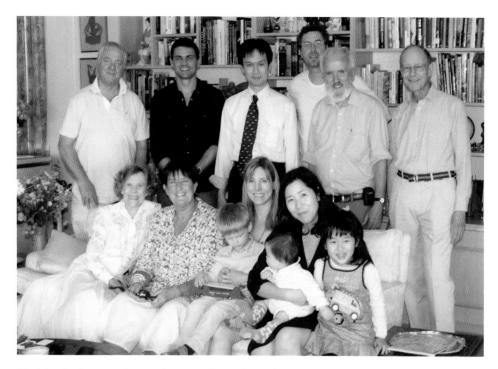

The Menière's research group host a welcome lunch for their Japanese research fellow, Yasuhiro 'Yas' Chihara, at the Kirkpatricks' apartment in Sydney, 3 April 2011. Back row from left: Bill Gibson, Daniel Brown, Yas Chihara, Stephen Spring, Ian Curthoys and Bruce Kirkpatrick. Front row from left: Juliet Kirkpatrick, Alex Gibson, Caroline Spring, with Alexander on her lap, Yoshie Chihara, with baby Hiroko on her lap, and Noriko sitting next to her.

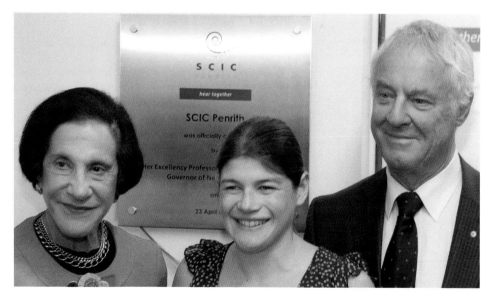

The Governor of NSW, Professor Marie Bashir, was the guest of honour at the official opening of the SCIC Penrith, which caters for clients in western Sydney and beyond, 23 April 2013. To the right of Professor Bashir is elite runner and cochlear implant recipient, Melinda Vernon from Springwood in the Blue Mountains, and Bill.

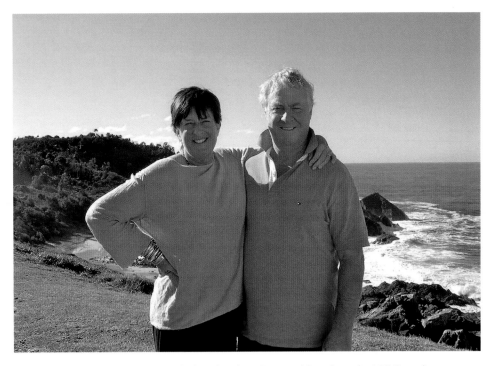

Bill and Alex enjoy leisure time with their family at Diamond Beach on the NSW north coast.

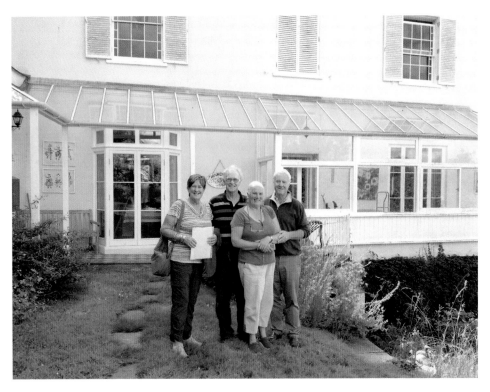

After both turning 70, Bill and Alex visited the home where he was born in Totnes and met the current owners of Lakemead, Julia and Nigel Kelland, June 2014.

rung her sister in Texas to enquire about having a cochlear implant in the US. 'We were told that one of the best men in the world was Professor Gibson – so we looked him up in the phone book.'[3]

The same week as he performed the surgery on Andreas, Bill operated on David Carter, who was now seven. When Bill had previously met David's mother Glenda at the Shepherd Centre, he told her that David was unsuitable for a cochlear implant due to his Mondini Syndrome, in which there is a limited number of turns in the cochlea. The syndrome, combined with dyspraxia, a problem in the brain's speech centre, had made it very difficult for David to learn to speak. He liked to draw as a means of communication, and this would later develop into a career as an animator.

During a more recent consultation about leakages of fluid from David's cochlea, Bill discovered that the boy had lost all his residual hearing and was experiencing continual dizzy spells. Bill suggested a cochlear implant and, after much soul-searching, Glenda told Bill they would go ahead, saying, 'If any surgeon can succeed in implanting a child with half a cochlea, it's you'.

On the day of David's five-hour operation, Glenda paced back and forth through the gardens of the Children's Hospital. When she saw Bill walking briskly towards her in his suit, she feared the worst. But then he called cheerfully over his shoulder, 'I'm just going to get another drill', and continued his brisk walk up the hill towards RPA. During David's switch-on at Chatswood PS, the Channel 9 news crew filmed his reaction to the flushing of the toilet at one end of the tiny storeroom. By rights, David's switch-on should have been performed in the brand new Yenibis Deafness Research Centre at the Children's Hospital, but Bill's dreams of a new centre for his young patients had turned to dust.

Hearing professionals from the PDSG had complained to John Yu that Bill had 'broken their embargo' by implanting progressively younger children. When the renovations at Wade House were completed, Yu was pressured by an inner circle of hearing professionals in the PDSG to allocate the space to the hospital audiologists. The floor plan and the equipment, designed by Christopher Game, were all tailored for the testing, fitting and programming of children with devices such as cochlear implants. Yu tried to convince the family of the late Arthur Yenibis that audiology was just as worthy a cause as cochlear implants, but they withdrew their donation. The hospital administration was not pleased, but Yu stood firm.[4] Bill was back to square one for the children's habilitation – 'a janitor's cupboard', as the Carter family had described it, at Chatswood PS.

* * *

The heart-warming photo of David Carter that appeared in the *Glebe Weekly* showed him with his arms around the shoulders of two much younger boys. The three of them are 'looking like little soldiers' because they each have bandages on their heads.[5] The headline above this article – 'Michael, David and Andreas are "$6m" kids' – is a reference to the 1970s television show *Six Million Dollar Man*, about an astronaut who had superhuman strength due to his bionic implants.

By the time Bill arrived in Australia in 1983, roughly this amount had already been invested in the Cochlear division of Paul Trainor's biotechnology holding company, Nucleus.[6] In 1988, Trainor decided to sell all six divisions of Nucleus to the Australian-owned company Pacific Dunlop because he was determined that his life's work should remain in Australian hands.[7] Bill says that the year before this sale, Paul Trainor had gone through a series of personal tragedies including the death of his son and his first wife. 'He gave away $30 million of the proceeds of the sale to his staff, various people working in the field and to selected charities.'[8]

Trainor was also very generous to Bill. For the CICADA Christmas gathering in 1988, Trainor offered to pay for a fully catered event at the Villa Maria school hall in Hunters Hill. There were clowns and stilt walkers to entertain the children, and Bill wore a padded suit to make the first of many appearances as Father Christmas. Despite feeling 'hot as Hades', Bill produced a present from his large sack for each child, only some of whom realised he was really their surgeon.

Early in 1989, Bill was present for the switch-on of his fiftieth cochlear implant recipient. A thirty-year-old woman named Paula experienced problems in the workplace when her House 3M implant completely broke down, so Bill performed an explant and replaced it with one of his publically funded Nucleus devices.[9] It was around this time that the American company 3M decided to withdraw from the cochlear implant market. In a costly exercise, but one that the CEO of the Cochlear division of Nucleus Ltd, David Money, believed to be ethically correct, the company took over the maintenance of the recipients who still had the House 3M device.[10]

Bill also made an expensive decision, which he believed to be in the interests of his youngest implant recipients, to rent a house near Chatswood PS for his children's implant program. Motivating factors were his frustration at having the Yenibis Centre taken away from him and the fact that his staff had run out of space. Prue Jeffrey realised one day that Bill was paying the rent out of his own pocket and says she will be 'eternally grateful to him for that'.

This two-bedroom Federation cottage was often referred to as 'Cochlear House' and not long after moving in Bill welcomed a visiting professor, Richard Tyler from Iowa University. An audiologist by training with a PhD in psychoacoustics, Tyler presented the findings of his independent assessment of the children at the first parent meeting in February 1989. He noted that the listening skills of the children in Bill's Sydney program were superior to those of children he had tested in other cochlear implant centres around the world.[11]

Bill had previously met Tyler in Bordeaux and their conversations about this renowned French wine region revived memories of the electrophysiology course he had attended at the Institut Georges Portmann in the 1970s. When Bill learned that Michel Portmann and his wife Claudine Portmann had accepted his invitation to lead some courses in Sydney, he wanted to give them a special treat. No doubt inspired by the 1988 bicentenary commemorations of the landing of the First Fleet, Bill booked a night for the French couple on board one of Captain Cook Cruises's tall ships for a sail down the Hawkesbury River. When Portman's audiologist René Dauman arrived instead of Claudine, Bill quickly organised two single beds and Dauman told Bill it was a great honour to share a cabin with his boss.

On 21 February 1989, a photo was taken at RPA of the forty or so participants fortunate enough to learn about electrocochleography and brainstem auditory evoked potentials from Michel Portmann, who was a founder of these techniques. Bill invited other 'celebrity' presenters from overseas to lead his three-day temporal bone workshops for ENT surgeons, including his friend David Moffat from Cambridge and Professors Meyerhoff, Marquet and Bebear. At the end of these courses a bottle of whisky was awarded to the ENT surgeon judged to have the most 'nimble fingers' for the bone dissection work and participants then enjoyed an evening of fine dining.

Professor Portmann contacted Bill and asked if a young French ENT specialist, Nicolas Guérin, could come to Sydney to gain some experience in the ENT department at RPA. Nicolas, who Bill recalls enjoyed surfing at Bondi Beach during his stay, was the first in a long line of fellows to join him from overseas. Following in Guérin's footsteps was Robert Gunn from Auckland, who had been recommended by Bill Baber, one of the surgeons Bill assisted in the first cochlear implant operation in New Zealand.

Having a fellow from overseas in his department was particularly useful at this time, because Bill had just lost his senior lecturer, Milton Waner, an expert in phototherapy in cancers. Bill's initial joy at finally being given a lecturer to assist him with his teaching load, including the medical students at the university, had turned to disappointment after only a year, when the funding for this position ran out. The University of Sydney wrote to inform Bill that there would be no replacement for Waner.[12] The following year, the funding also ran out for Christopher Game, whose official title was the Elizabeth Scott Fellow in Hearing Research. The only positive to come from Game's departure was that Bill would form a very close working relationship with Halit Sanli, a Turkish-born electrical and biomedical engineer who had previously worked as an oil extraction engineer in the North Sea.

* * *

While Barry Scrivener was undoubtedly the most helpful of the ENT specialists who had assisted Bill since his arrival in Australia, another guiding light during this time was Professor John Ward. Despite suffering severe bilateral hearing loss, Ward had risen through the ranks of Sydney University to his current role of vice-chancellor. Ward had established Bill's professorial chair through one donation of $250000 from Sir William Tyree and a second of the same amount from an anonymous donor.[13] Ward was currently providing invaluable assistance with the registration through the university senate of a new fundraising body, the EAR (Ear and Allied Research) Foundation, which would assume responsibility for the payment of the rent and other expenses for the cottage in Chatswood.

The ABC 702 presenter Margaret Throsby agreed to be a member of the media committee of the EAR Foundation and assisted Bill by inviting him to appear on her radio program. Bill recalls 'pleading his lot' for a two-year-old boy named Callum, who needed a cochlear implant. After the live interview, a couple rang the radio station and pledged $15000. When Bill asked them, 'What made you do it?', they explained that they were on the way to a furniture store when they heard his appeal on the radio. 'We can do without the lounge suite,' the couple told him, 'but Callum needs his hearing.' With the help of Rosalie Yaremko, who had recently arrived from Canada to join Bill's habilitation team, the guttural sounds that Callum had previously made slowly evolved into words such as 'up', 'more' and 'home'.

Bill didn't like to turn a single deaf child away from his program, so he considered it 'an absolute tragedy' that Felicity and Joseph Formosa had been made to wait so long for their cochlear implants. In 1989, their situation became even more urgent when it was realised that the sister and brother both suffered from the worst form of Usher Syndrome. The siblings' eyesight was deteriorating to the degree that their ability to use Sign Language was under threat and Bill was finally granted Ethics Committee approval to go ahead with their operations. He launched an urgent appeal for donors to come forward in the *Daily Mirror* and the Formosa family referred to him in this article as 'a genius with a kind heart'.[14] During her switch-on, eight-year-old Felicity was asked to describe the feeling of sound and used Sign Language to explain it was 'soft, different, better and special'. Bill knew that Felicity was a little too old to receive the full benefit of her implant and was frustrated that she had not been able to have the operation two years earlier, around the same time as Holly McDonell and Pia Jeffrey.

Pia was currently receiving daily therapy from her mother and a variety of teachers, including Sister Caterina Heffernan, a Catholic nun who Bill says worked in an honorary capacity with the deaf children, because 'teaching was her calling'. Pia's progress had been mentioned in a grant application. The local member for Willoughby and the Minister for Health, Peter Collins, visited Cochlear House for a morning tea because he wanted to meet the children and their parents. In July 1989, Collins announced $377 000 in state government funding, which would pay for the salaries of all staff at the house, plus equipment and free implants for families in need.

Until Bill received this 'enhancement grant', the entire upkeep of the house at Chatswood and its equipment had been paid for by the EAR Foundation, which had pledged ongoing support. Bill was very excited when he heard that the Governor-General, Bill Hayden, had accepted the invitation to be the guest of honour at a gala dinner to launch the EAR Foundation in mid-1990.[15]

Bill had been approached by the president of the Royal Institute for Deaf and Blind Children (RIDBC), Sir Garfield Barwick, about relocating the children's cochlear implant program to the RIDBC's new school for hearing- and sight-impaired children in North Parramatta. Even though Bill wasn't prepared to relinquish his program, he was happy to provide training for a teacher from the RIDBC at Cochlear House. Bill's habilitation staff also provided training for the preschool staff from the Shepherd Centre and hearing professionals from both the National Acoustic Laboratories and the NSW Department of Education, which had softened its stance against the children's cochlear implant program in recent times.

No one likes to lose a staff member who has made a valuable contribution to the establishment of a groundbreaking clinical program. However, the good working relationship between one of the members of the habilitation team and Bill, as well as the other staff members and the parents who attended sessions with their children, broke down irrevocably during the second half of 1989.

Some families were upset because they believed that this staff member (who Bill has been careful not to name in any discussions of this period) hadn't communicated problems relating to the functioning of their children's cochlear implants to the rest of the team.

Prue Jeffrey organised a meeting to tell Bill that her son Alex was not receiving the same clear signal through his speech processor as his older sister Pia, and would become distressed by the low whine of their washing machine. Bill decided to replace Alex's implant. A distraught Glenda and Garth Carter came to Bill's home in Wahroonga for a private meeting one evening, because their son David said that activation of certain electrodes in his implant felt like 'raw nerve pain'. A solution was found when Bill suggested they visit the audiologist at the Cochlear division of Nucleus Ltd to have some of David's electrodes switched off – just like Charles Pauka had once done for Alan Jones at RPA.

The period surrounding the breakdown of the relationship and subsequent departure of the team member concerned was extremely stressful for everyone involved with the program. The consensus among the staff and parents was that it was preferable for her not to return. The primary concern of Bill and his team was that the children did not suffer as a result of the dispute.

The staff member commenced legal action but eventually she formally resigned from the Children's Hospital. John Yu had been very supportive of Bill during this period. Bill was very pleased that the friendly, cooperative atmosphere returned to the house in Chatswood and he wrote to John Yu in April 1990 that he hoped 'the unfortunate affair' was now behind them.

One Sunday in late May of that same year, Bill and his family heard a great number of ambulances wailing past their Wahroonga home. An intercity express train had smashed into the last carriage of a historic locomotive, killing and injuring members of a group of day-trippers from the University of Sydney who a newspaper article described as sharing 'a passion and love for steam trains'.[16] Bill was saddened to discover that among the six pronounced dead were the recently retired John Ward, his wife Patricia and their eldest daughter, 36-year-old Jennifer.

Only weeks after the death of this great mentor, Bill was disturbed to find two auditors sitting outside his office in the Blackburn Building. They told him that he had been accused of misappropriating EAR Foundation funds. The staff and the parents of the children's cochlear implant program were shocked to learn that this was the result of allegations made by the former team member.

* * *

On 29 June 1990, Bill asked his secretary Joan Lehane to send urgent faxes to both the deputy vice-chancellor of the university, Professor Michael Taylor, and the president of the EAR Foundation, Sir William Tyree, requesting their assistance. A major independent enquiry was set up under Professor James McLeod and during the next four months Bill had to account for all his actions and every dollar he had spent. He said, '[I felt] fairly secure as I had never even claimed a bus fare from the EAR Foundation.'[17] He knew that if he had inadvertently made an error he could have lost his job and would probably have needed to return to England.

Bill felt compelled to cancel the dinner to launch the foundation, because of complaints made to the Independent Commission Against Corruption (ICAC) and the Ombudsman. He sent the following letter to all concerned: 'I regret that a cloud covers the EAR Foundation and until this has been investigated and cleared, it would be unfair to the Governor-General of the Commonwealth of Australia or any of our supporters to continue with the dinner.'

Not long after this letter was sent, Bill received a beautiful letter of support signed by the parents of nineteen children attending Cochlear House: 'We have no doubts that any review of these matters will prove baseless. Accordingly, we take this opportunity to confirm our full faith and support for you in ALL your actions so far and in the future.' It wasn't only the parents who rallied around Bill. Some of his staff from Cochlear House helped to collate the administrative records and patient files for the investigation. They didn't want the door closed on what lay in store for these deaf children and their families.

It was a great pity that John Ward never heard the very welcome news that Bill had been completely exonerated by the ICAC enquiry and told he was 'the squeakiest clean professor in the University'.[18] The auditors had even found some EAR Foundation funds in another university bank account and transferred them back. Bill's biggest fear during what he describes as 'this horrendous period, for both myself and Alex' was that the NSW Minister for Health would remove his annual grant for cochlear implants. Then he would have had to go back to relying on donations from benefactors, giving talks in shopping centres and making appeals in the newspapers. One of the fallouts of the accusations and resulting legal action was that Bill had not been able to perform cochlear implant surgery on any children for most of 1990.

One of the children awaiting surgery was a girl whose computed tomography (CT) scan revealed that her cochlea was filled with bony growth, due to a previous meningitis infection. In December 1990 Bill performed what he called an 'inlay' procedure on this girl, which involved drilling out a channel in her cochlea, from the round window opening to the first basal turn. This landmark operation allowed him to place five electrodes inside her cochlea.[19] Bill repeated the procedure on other children, including a four-year-old boy; managing to insert fifteen electrodes into his cochlea.[20] From then on he advocated that children have a cochlear implant operation within a year of their meningitis infection, so that there was less opportunity for the pus in their cochlear duct to harden into bone.

All of the children with acquired deafness who had received a cochlear implant in the program to date, including the first child, Holly McDonell, had been deafened by meningitis. When Holly was around eight years old, she volunteered to help on the CICADA stand at the Hearing Expo, held during Hearing Awareness Week at the State Library in Macquarie Street, Sydney. Bill recalls that a Signing Deaf couple turned up at the stand and, through an interpreter, asked her, 'Does your cochlear implant hurt, little girl?' Holly looked up at Bill and he could tell that she thought it was a crazy question. He was careful not to react in any way because he was trying desperately to make peace with the Signing Deaf community.

During Hearing Awareness Week an article appeared in the *Sydney Morning Herald* about whether all deaf children should learn the Australian Sign Language, Auslan.[21] When interviewed for the article, Renee Hardy said that her six-year-old daughter Amelia knew a little Sign Language and when she was older could decide for herself if she wanted to use it. The same article mentioned that when Amelia had her implant at two years and ten months, she had a vocabulary of ten words, but now, three or four years later, her spoken vocabulary was about 2000 words.

Bill attributed such a dramatic post-implant improvement to 'brain plasticity', which was at this time a relatively new area of research, pioneered by Michael Merzenich and some of his colleagues in the US.[22] Bill says that the greater the importance of an ability – for example, sight, hearing or movement – to our survival, the shorter the period that the brain will remain 'plastic'. In an article Bill wrote for the *Medical Journal of Australia*, he stated, 'It is likely that the ability of the human brain to learn sounds completely naturally is lost by the age of two years. If the deaf child is given a hearing aid or cochlear implant after this age, the acquisition of listening (and speech) is no longer natural and the child has to be taught "every inch of the way".[23]

Pia Jeffrey is an example of such a child. After receiving a cochlear implant and several years of intense habilitation she had been transformed into an extremely talkative child. Pia was fortunate to have the implant when this outstanding result was still possible, and her face would soon grace the back cover of the Sydney telephone directory to promote the Australian bionic ear. Bill comments that if someone brought a congenitally deaf six-year-old child to him for a cochlear implant assessment today he would probably tell them, 'You've left it a bit late'.

The FDA had by now approved the bionic ear as being 'safe and effective for use in children from two to eighteen years of age'[24] and in the years ahead Bill would operate on children at incrementally younger ages; even those younger than two. The habilitation these toddlers required was reduced to around three to six months as they learnt sounds 'naturally' in normal family situations.

At CICADA's Christmas luncheon, Bill wore his black academic robes from the University of London to add a sense of importance to the occasion as he presented certificates to the children who were moving on to other centres or to 'big school'. After lunch a photo was taken of Bill with Felicity and Joseph Formosa, who were seated on either side of him, looking happy and ready for their summer holidays.

With the money left to him by his mother, Bill purchased a block of land in a new housing estate at Diamond Beach, on the NSW north coast. The two-storey wooden holiday house constructed on this land would provide a base for Bill and Alex to enjoy leisure time with their grown-up children – Laura, who was in the final stages of a physiotherapy degree, and Hugh, who had commenced business studies since returning from a Rotary exchange year to Brazil.

The storm clouds had finally parted. When a former boss from the London Hospital, Peter McKelvie, visited Bill in Sydney, he could see that he had made a good life for himself in Australia. McKelvie said, 'Look, Bill, you're probably no longer interested but Professor Don Harrison's job has come up at Gray's Inn Road.' Bill told him, 'I don't need a fall-back plan. I'm staying put.' Few would have realised how close Australia came to losing a cochlear implant surgeon who ranks among our finest and certainly our most prolific.

CHAPTER 11

Casting the net long and wide

**He implanted kids from south-east
Asia who came to Australia with their
families as part of the overseas program,
so the net from Prof is cast long and wide.**

Shaun Hand, general manager of Cochlear
Australia and New Zealand

When the lights dimmed at the after-dinner meeting of the
Northampton Medical Society, the first slide was not the one
Bill was expecting. It showed him diving bare-bottomed into a
stream near Argelès-sur-Mer and brought back memories of the
camping holidays he and his sister's families had enjoyed together in
the early 1980s. His brother-in-law Richard Marshall had slipped
the slide into the carousel as an ice-breaker for Bill's talk, 'Deaf children and cochlear implants' – a controversial topic in the United
Kingdom, because few children had yet received the cochlear

device. Eleanor had never heard Bill speak in public before and said, 'Even as his sister, I could not help but be transfixed'.

Bill relished the opportunity to connect with small groups such as the forty or so doctors he addressed in Northampton. At the other end of the scale were the lectures he gave at conferences, such as the British Academic Conference of Otolaryngology (BACO) and the American Academy of Otolaryngology – Head and Neck Surgeons, which both attracted audiences in the thousands.

These conferences were important for making professional contacts, such as the celebrated American otologist John Shea Jr, with whom Bill shared late-night telephone conversations about their respective theories on the cause of Menière's disease. After attending the Shambaugh–Shea Weekend of Otology in 1992 they travelled from Chicago on to Memphis, where John Shea Jr had been inducted into the Hall of Fame on the same day as Elvis Presley. Bill visited the four-storey Shea Clinic, where he observed Shea performing the stapedectomy operation he first performed in 1956 to successfully restore the hearing of a woman with conductive hearing loss.[1]

Although some Australian colleagues viewed his attendance at these overseas meetings as self-promotion, Bill believed that he was promoting the standing of Australian otolaryngology and what would become the jewel in its crown: the bionic ear. During talks about his children's cochlear implant program Bill showed videos of paediatric recipients, including Holly McDonell regaining her speech in sessions conducted at home by her mother Viktorija.

As a result of these presentations, Bill received hundreds of requests each year from medical and allied health professionals from around the world to meet his habilitation team in Sydney. However, this team would soon need to find a new home, due to a crisis with their rented premises in Chatswood. Their neighbours in Anderson Street had complained to the Willoughby council about 'a brothel in their midst'. Bill went to the council chambers to explain that the young women coming and going from the house were actually mothers dropping off their preschool-aged children. The mayor of Willoughby, Greg Bartels, was sympathetic and guided Bill through this item at the next council meeting. Bartels also assisted Bill with all the paperwork necessary to help him find properly licensed premises.

When Bill and his staff moved into a three-bedroom Federation house at 246A Willoughby Road, Naremburn, they acquired a new name – the Children's Cochlear Implant Centre (CCIC) – and a new logo in the form of Sidney the snail. Line drawings of this cute character appeared on banners, the white T-shirts worn by the children and the cake Alex Gibson ordered especially for the official opening of the centre. To amuse the children, Bill started wearing ties adorned with snails and bright yellow socks, which have been trademark items of his wardrobe ever since.

On 17 August 1992 the NSW Minister for Health Ron Phillips unveiled the centre's name plaque. Phillips had brought his parents with him to the opening, and Bill noticed that they both communicated by finger spelling – a form of Sign Language where each letter is spelt out. The Channel 7 news team filmed Ron Phillips with John Yu and several of the children in the back garden of the house, next to a bright yellow marquee.

A journalist covering the opening of the new centre asked Bill to comment on the opposition he had faced to his children's implant program. Bill replied that the cochlear implant was as revolutionary as the hearing aid. 'When Alexander Graham Bell invented the hearing aid, they (Signing Deaf people) thought he was the devil incarnate.'[2] Not much had changed because Bill recalls attending meetings where members of the Deaf community would make the sign for 'devil' as he entered the room, by holding two fingers above their heads to depict the devil's horns.

One of the many letters Bill received criticising him for performing surgery on the congenitally deaf child Pia Jeffrey was from a former UK colleague, Graham Fraser, who was the president of the British Cochlear Implant Group. After hearing Bill's talk at a BACO meeting in Dublin, Graham and his wife Patricia requested a visit to the CCIC. A child who made a particular impression on the English guests was four-year-old Jacob 'Jake' Fisher. Jake was born congenitally deaf and had an expressive vocabulary of nil at the time of his cochlear implant operation two years before. Graham Fraser asked him, 'Did you come here today by motorcar?', which Bill points out is a very English way of asking the question. With his teacher and mother sitting by his side, Jake answered confidently, 'No, I flew here by plane this morning. We live really far away!'[3]

Graham Fraser was so impressed by this interaction with Jake that he organised a follow-up visit to the centre by a consultant he knew from Cambridge, Roger Gray. At the encouragement of Graham Fraser and John Graham from University College Hospital (UCH) in London, Roger Gray had become a member of the UCH Implant Group and performed cochlear implant operations on children with acquired deafness, including the first child in the UK to receive a cochlear implant. When he visited Sydney in 1992, Gray was interested to see the results Bill was achieving with the Nucleus device on congenitally deaf children and commented, 'I've never seen or heard of anything better than the work that's being done here'.[4]

The CCIC attracted world-wide interest during 1993, with 300 international visitors from countries including the UK, Sweden, the US, South America, New Zealand, Hong Kong, Taiwan, Japan, Thailand, Korea and Indonesia. These visits no doubt provided inspiration and confidence for other cochlear implant programs, as it had for Roger Gray with his paediatric program at Addenbrooke's Hospital in Cambridge, where Bill's friend David Moffat also worked.

Lady Pauline Ashley and her husband, Lord Jack Ashley of Stoke – a couple who Bill knew from London – sought his advice about cochlear implants during 1993. Lord Ashley had been deafened as a complication of ear surgery, so he was understandably feeling apprehensive about having another ear operation. During a visit to Sydney they had breakfast at a hotel in the city with Alex and Bill, who organised a meeting with Alan Jones, a cochlear implant recipient of a similar age. Lord Ashley returned to the UK very enthusiastic about having a cochlear implant.

Bill and his UK colleagues were saddened to hear that only three months after performing this surgery, Graham Fraser died at the age of fifty-seven, in February 1994. Lord Ashley played an important role in establishing the Graham Fraser Memorial Foundation, which raised the funds for an Otology Fellowship. Bill would later feel honoured to be chosen as the only surgeon who would be training these fellows. Lord Ashley's correspondence with Bill included a story about a visit to a pond with his three-year-old grandson, where they noticed insects skimming the surface. Ashley was thrilled to be able to hear Harry tell him, 'They're not flies, Grandad'.

* * *

Many of the recipients in Bill's children's implant program were currently hovering around two years of age, the lower age limit recommended by the FDA. Bill stated in a paper he presented at an Audiological Society of Australia meeting, 'We feel it is no longer reasonable for us to exclude children under two from receiving a cochlear implant, especially in view of the enormous potential for their success.' The first child to break this age barrier in Australia, and possibly the world, was Teigan van Roosmalen.[5] When Bill first performed ECochG testing on Teigan to assess her suitability for a cochlear implant, she was only sixteen months old and he told her mother, 'She's one of the deafest little girls I've seen, but she's still too young'.

Bill used a modified version of the ECochG test on Teigan which he had developed with the assistance of his biomedical engineer Halit Sanli and his Japanese fellow Shin Aso.[6] Previously Bill pointed a wire probe towards the round window entrance to the cochlea, which he noted could be a bit 'hit and miss'. For the modified ECochG test, Bill asked Halit to solder the metal wire into a 'golf club' shape, which fits snugly into a niche of the round window, like a fist in a baseball glove. Bill considers the 'golf club' to be an important contribution to the field of electrophysiology.

When Teigan van Roosmalen was twenty months old, Bill met with his team and they all agreed that she would benefit from a cochlear implant. He sought approval from the Ethics Committee at the Children's Hospital and Teigan's operation would be the first he performed at the new Mater Hospital in Rocklands Road, Crows Nest. On the day of her switch-on, Teigan kept turning her head towards the audiologist, wondering where the sound was coming from. To her parents' delight, her frustration levels, behaviour and vocal sounds all soon improved.

It is possible for children as young as Teigan to have a cochlear implant because the cochlea is adult sized at birth. Bill then performed the surgery on an even younger child: seventeen-month-old 'Little' John Erdman Jr from Scone, who believes that he was the first Aboriginal child to receive a cochlear implant. The wall plaque presented to Bill by the Erdman family, which is in the shape of Australia and features the Aboriginal flag, still hangs on the wall outside his office today.

The CCIC was now assisting between forty and sixty families each year from all over New South Wales. The team even accepted into the program a little boy named Rick from Tully in far north Queensland, whose family stayed in Bill and Alex's backyard cabana during his habilitation. Bill also received letters from families who lived in countries neighbouring Australia which did not yet have their own cochlear implant programs. Shaun Hand – who in a few years' time would be appointed general manager of Cochlear Australia and New Zealand – said, 'He implanted kids from south-east Asia who came to Australia with their families as part of the overseas program, so the net from Prof is cast long and wide'. Two of the first overseas children to receive cochlear implants as part of this program were Karim from Malaysia and Anna from Indonesia, whose families moved to Sydney for six to twelve months during 1993. Anna, who was about eighteen, was the daughter of an Indonesian general and after her return home featured on the cover of a women's magazine.

Over the next couple of years, Bill would perform cochlear implant operations on approximately forty children from countries in south-east Asia. A new entity was created, Cochlear Implants International (CII), which employed hearing professionals including: Colleen Psarros, Rosalie Yaremko, William Woytowych, Colleen Everingham and Andrew Kendrick. The director of CII was Judy Wimble, who had previously held administrative roles with both the children's cochlear implant program and the EAR Foundation.

Nine-year-old John Lui was living with his Australian-Chinese family in Hong Kong, at the northern end of Lantau Island, when he caught the flu and lost his small amount of residual hearing. When his mother, Sandra Lui, spoke to Judy Wimble she learnt the good news that Bill had started an overseas program and brought John to Sydney for testing. John can remember Bill being very jovial before his cochlear implant operation to help him relax.

The Lui family lived in Sydney during John's post-implant habilitation, but afterwards they returned to Hong Kong, where John's father worked. John's family were delighted to learn that as private clients of CII, his after-implant care included visits by the audiologist Colleen Psarros. Soon members of the CII team would be flying to Asia three times a year for the habilitation of the overseas children, working either in English or the child's first language.

The families in the overseas program were encouraged to join in with the activities of the CCIC. This included a parents' weekend residential workshop organised by Teigan's mother Dee van Roosmalen at the Naamaroo Convention Centre at Lane Cove River Park, with Bill as one of the guest speakers. Victorija McDonell was very active in organising fundraising events to purchase Christmas presents for the children and she certainly pulled some strings to secure the services of the Australian rock group Mental as Anything to appear at Moby Dick's restaurant in Whale Beach.

At the annual CICADA Christmas luncheon for cochlear implant recipients, which Paul Trainor was still funding, approximately one-hundred children sat in a semi-circle on the parquetry floor of the Villa Maria school hall to watch the magic show and receive a bag of presents and novelty items from Santa. The children were confused when they saw Bill standing next to someone dressed in a Santa suit who was nearly identical in appearance. Even the most recent of the audiologists to join the adult cochlear implant program at RPA, Monica Bray, did a double take as she had never met Bob before.

Monica Bray, with her slight German–Brazilian accent, was making her mark on the adult cochlear implant program. She had earned the title 'the matchmaker' because she ensured that everyone had at least one 'implant buddy' of a similar age and background. As the number of implant recipients started to rise exponentially, Monica wrote protocols to ensure that the patients all received the same high level of service and care. She spent her weekends photocopying information packs for both patients and professionals in the audiology team's dark and musty new premises, which they referred to as 'the dungeon'. Since losing their little corner of the

Brown Street Outpatients Department, they had moved to some below-ground-level rooms in RPA's former resident medical officer (RMO) quarters, located on a driveway running along the rear of the hospital. This driveway forms the boundary between the hospital and the University of Sydney.

Next to the old RMO's quarters was the equally historic former nurses' accommodation, which Bill sometimes used as a short-cut to the hospital's operating theatres from his office in the university. One day he found yellow tape across the door marked: 'Do Not Enter'. Ignoring the warning, he ventured into the maze of dark passageways and soon realised he was lost. 'There were these two ladies who pointed the way out,' says Bill, who noticed that the women were dressed in floor-length Victorian nurses' uniforms identical to those displayed on mannequins in the entrance foyer of RPA. The building was demolished soon after this spooky experience and Bill asked himself, 'Were they ghosts?'

* * *

The first of Bill's patients to receive the Nucleus device, Sue Walters, still visited the implant team at RPA on a regular basis for speech testing as well as mapping and upgrades of her speech processor. Her cochlear implant had inspired her to study for a Bachelor of Science and just before her final exams in 1994, Sue and her husband Wayne became parents, three weeks earlier than expected, to a baby girl, Ruby.

Sue says her science degree gave her a greater appreciation of the 'sheer dedication and hard work' of pioneers of the bionic ear, including Graeme Clark in Melbourne and Jim Patrick at the Cochlear division of Nucleus Ltd. Many admired the way David Money's replacement as the CEO of this division, Catherine Livingstone, steered the company's acquisition from Pacific Dunlop before it was launched onto the Australian stock exchange in 1995.[7] Pacific Dunlop sold the other divisions to foreign interests, so Cochlear Ltd was the only one to remain Australian-owned.[8] Before the float, Bill was offered 2000 shares at the listing price of $2.50 each, but declined because he considered it to be a conflict of interest for a surgeon to recommend a company's products and then benefit from an increase in its profits.

That offer would have represented a considerable sum at today's listed price for Cochlear shares, but money has never been a motivating factor during Bill's medical career. Some cochlear implant surgeons charge thousands of dollars on top of the rebate private patients receive from their private care health fund, but Bill has never charged a 'gap' since arriving in Australia. He says, 'I've never felt the need'.

The 2UE radio host Stan Zemanek considered that people like Bill who help others every day are more deserving of 'gongs' such as the Australian of the Year award than members of rock bands. After their radio interview, Zemanek sent a letter to Bill stating that his work with cochlear implant patients deserved all the recognition it could receive, 'and judging by the reaction of our listeners, you are to be commended'.

Some members of the Rotary Club of Berowra were clearly thinking along the same lines as Zemanek, because they secretly nominated Bill for an Australian of the Year award. The nomination paper, which described Bill as a 'mild mannered, unassuming, almost retiring man', resulted in his receiving a general division award (AM) from the Governor-General Bill Hayden. After the story of his AM award half-filled the front page of the *Hornsby and Upper North Shore Advocate*,[9] Bill wrote a letter to the editor saying: 'I was very flattered to get my award, although I am not sure that I deserve it. My success is only due to all those who have given me so much help. I have had marvellous support from colleagues … and the dedication of the staff at the Children's Cochlear Implant Centre has been the most important factor in the success of the program.'[10]

Equally unexpected was the Variety Club's Humanitarian Award, which was presented to Bill at a black-tie dinner in 1994 at the Sheraton-Wentworth Hotel where he met the winners of other Heart Awards, including the gardening show host Don Burke and the Australian singer of Malaysian extraction Kamahl. Five months after this awards night, Bill received a letter from the club president, Tony Hasham, stating: 'I am delighted to formally advise you that the Variety Club of Australia has approved a grant of $737 000 for the purpose of building and furnishing a new centre on a site yet to be determined in metropolitan Sydney.'

This was the largest single donation Bill had ever been pledged. The letter confirming the amount was presented to him on the Doug Mulray Show one Saturday evening, in front of a live audience at the Channel 7 studios. Some of the children and parents from the CCIC were in the studio audience and after the show a photo was taken of Doug Mulray and Bill standing on either side of a piano with nine-year-old Amelia Hardy sitting on the top.

It had been Bill's long-held dream to provide a permanent centre for the children's cochlear implant program. Bert Hely, the chairman of the EAR Foundation, was a practising architect and offered to take on the role of designing a purpose-built centre. Some vacant land on the perimeter of Concord Hospital was floated by a NSW state politician as a possible location, and Hely set to work immediately on the plans.

Even though Hely's offer would potentially save many thousands of dollars, a major fundraising drive was planned to ensure the EAR Foundation would be able to see the project through to completion. It was hoped that a Christmas Appeal collection box at the Chatswood Chase shopping centre would raise $10 000. Some of Bill's paediatric implant recipients went up on stage at the shopping centre before the performance of *A Christmas Carol*, including fourteen-month-old Sally Wiltshire-Bridle, who was in her mother's arms.

Another fundraiser was the East–West Ball, which was hosted for several years in a row by Lady Mary Fairfax, the third wife and widow of Sir Warwick Fairfax, in a marquee erected on the front lawn of her home, Fairwater, in Sydney's eastern suburbs. The proceeds from the ball were split equally between the Opera Foundation and the children's cochlear implant program.

One year Bill took as his guest ten-year-old Callum, who had received his implant at the age of three after an ABC 702 radio appeal raised the money for his Nucleus device. Bill and Callum rubbed shoulders with guests such as Prince Albert of Monaco and Bob Hawke, the former Australian prime minister. Hawke, who served as PM from 1983 to 1991, picked up on Bill's English accent and asked him, 'When did you come to Australia?' When Bill told him 1983, Hawke said, 'Oh, just in time for the golden years'.

Bill and Bob were both busy with their respective careers and only saw each other about half a dozen times a year, but they have always liked to celebrate their birthdays together. For their combined 'hundredth' birthday celebration, the brothers enjoyed a lunch with close friends and family at the restaurant occupying the historic Banjo Patterson's Cottage in Gladesville, which overlooks the water.

A topic of conversation at the lunch was the fiftieth anniversary of the D-day landings in Normandy. Bob and Jan had just returned from the commemoration ceremonies in France, which they had attended with John and Eleanor. The symmetrical rows of white crosses reminded John of his great war-time friends Craven and Watty, who never made it off Sword Beach on 6 June 1944. Bill encouraged his father to write an account of the six years he served as a medical officer during World War II, so the stories of his bravery could be read by his grandchildren and great-grandchildren.

* * *

By mid-1994, Bill and his surgical colleagues had performed cochlear implant operations on more than one-hundred children and one-hundred and fifteen adults. For over a decade they had used a 20-centimetre, C-shaped incision, similar in size to that used by surgeons in Melbourne and other cochlear implant programs around the world. Typically, these large surgical incisions took several weeks to heal.[11] Bill and his co-surgeon at the Children's Hospital, Henley Harrison, noticed that blood sometimes collected under the large flap of skin, causing the wound to break down, and patients complained of numbness and pain along the edges of the incision. The worst-case scenario was for the implanted device to protrude through the flap – particularly in very young and very old implant recipients.

Bill gradually decreased the size of his incision until it was a straight vertical line measuring only 7 centimetres in length. The position of the new incision is close behind the recipient's ear and the surgeon places the disc-shaped implant into a tight pocket of connective tissue, where it remains firmly in place without the need for Dacron ties. In an initial clinical trial of twenty adults and thirty-two children, Bill found that the wound healed in only a few days and the infection rate was practically zero.[12] Many surgeons were sceptical at first about Bill's small, straight incision, but it was popularised overseas by surgeons including Gerry O'Donoghue from Nottingham and is now widely used around the world.

When the Children's Hospital moved from Camperdown to Westmead in western Sydney, the heritage façade of the main building was the only reminder of its former existence. The first operation Bill performed at the New Children's Hospital at Westmead, as it was called for many years, was on two-year-old Si Yuan, who spoke only Cantonese and was taught in her mother tongue, like some of the children from the overseas program.

Interestingly, the switch-on of Si Yuan took place the same month Bill was invited to deliver the Dr Li Dak Sum Shanghai–Hong Kong Development Lecture in the mainly Cantonese-speaking city of Hong Kong. During this visit to Hong Kong in December 1994, Bill performed cochlear implant surgeries with Professor Andrew van Hasselt on two adult patients at the Prince of Wales Hospital.[13] These were the early days in the use of the Nucleus device in both Hong Kong and mainland China, where the first two patients were implanted five months later at the Peking Union Hospital in Beijing in May 1995.[14]

Bill made travel plans for India for what promised to be two equally historic operations with Sandra Desa Souza, and collected the free implants from the Cochlear headquarters. Just as he was about to board the plane, Bill heard that Sandra's husband had accepted the franchise for the Austrian brand of implant, MED-EL. Bill went ahead with the trip, where he delivered the 1996 annual oration in memory of Sandra's father, Joe De Sa, in Lonavala and then travelled to Mumbai, which he describes as 'total chaos', to demonstrate the cochlear implant surgery to Sandra Desa Souza.

Some people considered it a strange way to relax in the evenings, but Bill spent hours watching videos of difficult cochlear implant surgeries to establish ways in which they could be improved and made more routine. He considered himself fortunate to be able to operate during his career alongside some of the world's leading cochlear implant surgeons, including Professor Jorge Schwartzman from Buenos Aires, who, in 1987, was the first surgeon in Latin America to perform a multichannel cochlear implant operation.[15] During Bill's visit to the British Hospital in Buenos Aires, he operated alongside Schwartzman, which provided an opportunity for him to discuss the stages in the development of his new surgical incision.

* * *

Bill and Alex had formed a close association with the family of one of the children in the overseas program, Iskandar Alsagoff, from Ipoh in Malaysia. Iskandar was six years old when Bill performed his cochlear implant surgery in February 1995. After his switch-on, Iskandar was integrated into a Year 2 class at a private boys' school in Sydney's eastern suburbs. During the family's stay in Sydney, Bill remembers having chilli mud crab in a restaurant with Iskandar's mother, Princess Nazhatul Shima (popularly known as Dottie), whose father was the former Sultan of Perak. 'Alex and I were absolutely covered [in spicy sauce], but Dottie didn't have a speck on her. She wasn't even wearing a bib,' says Bill in amazement.

In January 1996, Princess Dottie brought Iskandar back to Sydney for his one-year check-up with the habilitation team at the CCIC. The family gave Bill a newspaper clipping from the 17 January 1996 edition of the *New Straits Times*, which showed Iskandar meeting the wife of the Australian prime minister, Annita Keating, on her visit to the ENT department of the Universiti Kebangsaan Malaysia in Kuala Lumpur.[16] A sixteen-year-old boy in the same photo was the first person to have had cochlear implant surgery in Malaysia; however, this local implant program would have come too late for Iskandar. His parents have always been very grateful to Bill and Alex, who they would later invite to Iskandar's post-graduation ceremony after he completed a business degree at the University of New South Wales. During the years ahead, the overseas program would be disbanded as countries in south-east Asia began performing cochlear implant surgery on their own patients.

The CCIC was so short of space that Bill recalls his latest fellow, Neill Boustred, 'having to sit on the loo with his laptop computer perched on his knee'. Next to him in the bathroom, there were filing cabinets in the shower. Boustred had come from South Africa and is now an eminent ENT specialist in the northern Sydney suburb of Hornsby. Bill's previous fellow, Christopher Low, returned to Singapore, where he established a cochlear implant program and performed the first paediatric cochlear implant surgery in that country.

Rather than receiving fellows from a variety of countries, from January 1996 onwards Bill would host a fellow from the United Kingdom every year as part of the newly established Graham Fraser Memorial Fellowship. Two of the friends Bill trained with at the Middlesex Hospital, Jonathan Hazell and John Graham, became the trustees for this foundation, and John also interviewed potential candidates at his Harley Street rooms in London.

By the early months of 1996, Bill started to worry that time was running out to commence the building of their new premises using the Variety Club grant. He was informed by the area health executive that Concord Repatriation Hospital was unsuitable for such a venture because there was insufficient clinical support for the children. Bill could only surmise that the area executive did not want to approve any new buildings until a decision had been made on the proposed closure of Concord Hospital. Even if a suitable new site had now been identified, it was too late. In June 1996, Bill received a fax from the Chief Barker of the Variety Club to inform him that 'the current grant has been written back for accounting purposes and we invite you to re-apply when your organisation feels it appropriate'.[17] Bill recalls that Bert Hely was so upset about the project being 'canned' that he resigned as the chairman of the EAR Foundation.

It was a double blow for Bill to lose first the Yenibis Centre and now this grant of close to $750 000 for the construction of a new centre. Andrew Refshauge, the NSW Minister for Health and Aboriginal Affairs, allocated a wing of the Old Gladesville Hospital to Bill as temporary space for the children's cochlear implant program.[18] The architect's plans for the Yenibis Centre and the

proposed purpose-built centre at Concord Hospital only had about
five rooms each, but this temporary space was on two levels and in
Bill's mind seemed 'to stretch for miles'. They were only required to
pay a peppercorn rent of $1 per year and it was easy for Bill to
imagine the word 'temporary' soon being replaced with the word
'permanent'. Bill went home to tell Alex that the former psychiatric
wing was full of cobwebs and 'desperately in need of cheering
up' but it was the base they had hoped to find for the children's
implant program.

CHAPTER 12

A new centre and a new manager

[It was a relief] when into our lives
came young Christopher Rehn,
who arrived with such enthusiasm
and is another one who loves
and lives for the job.

Alex Gibson[1]

The first of two 'ups' that Bill can clearly remember from 1996 was being offered the space in a former women's psychiatric wing of the Old Gladesville Hospital. For the first few years, there were still some patients roaming around inside the hospital's high sandstone perimeter walls, including Elsie, who Bill recalls was tied to the waist of her minder by a cord, and a 'dear old man' who sat on the same seat all day long. The former hospital wing had missing floorboards downstairs which revealed a dank basement and holding rooms, to which patients had once been transported via an underground tunnel from the nearby 'Bedlam Wharf'. The cochlear implant program was responsible for the running costs of this historic sandstone building and for the renovations to make it a bit 'less creepy'.

The second 'up' was a new manager for the children's cochlear implant program. Twenty-seven-year-old Chris Rehn was interviewed by a panel at the New Children's Hospital at Westmead, which he thinks 'speaks of the joint ownership of the new centre by the Children's Hospital and the University of Sydney'. The first time Chris visited the Old Gladesville Hospital he met Alex Gibson, who had an old black Labrador trailing along behind her.

Alex was project managing the renovations of the centre with Doug Herridge, the husband of the family counsellor Susan Herridge. Initially these premises were so cavernous that Alex and Doug had to whistle to find each other. They received free building services from Tony Brown, the father of two children from Narrabri who had received cochlear implants, Maddelin and Liam. When the renovations were complete, Alex received many offers of assistance with decorations and furnishings to make it a welcoming place for the children.

Bill was very grateful to Andrew Refshauge, the NSW Minister for Health and Aboriginal Affairs, for the new premises and invited him to unveil the plaque at the official opening of the centre on 7 September 1996. Bill can remember Alex and Laura applying the last stencil of Sidney the snail to the fresh paintwork with less than half an hour to spare before the arrival of the official guests. For Bill, no party is complete without entertainment for the little ones, so he arranged for a giant, brightly coloured jumping castle to be set up in the grassy courtyard.

Now that Laura and Hugh were no longer living at home, Bill and Alex placed a deposit on a townhouse in a complex under construction which was only a fifteen-minute drive from the Old Gladesville Hospital. Laura lived in Gladesville with her husband

Stephen Begbie and their new baby, Jack. On one of their visits to see their first grandchild, Bill and Alex had their Labrador with them. Stephen, who worked as an oncologist at Royal North Shore Hospital, said to Bill, 'I think Bess has cancer'. Bill can clearly remember the distressing day when he and Alex took Bess to the veterinary surgery near their Wahroonga home to be put down. 'We were crying so much, the vet had to ask us to leave by the back door.'

Chris Rehn recalls that 'Prof and Alex opened up to me from day one'. He enjoyed discussions over impromptu dinners with his new boss and says that, 'Prof had complete faith in my abilities and never questioned if I was the right man for the job'. Chris had previously been 'burnt' in corporate health and found Bill's approach to finances 'refreshing'. Instead of building the business model first and the service delivery model second, Bill did the opposite. 'Prof was working to a cause and offered exactly the kind of low-cost model I wanted to see for our patients.'

For the eight staff members who came to Gladesville from the rented house in Naremburn, it was a lean exercise in the early days and they used a large, columned book to book appointments for the patients. Theresa Spraggon knew from personal experience about the hearing journey because her son Alex has a cochlear implant. Theresa's administrative and financial role evolved into one where she was able to form a close relationship with the children and their families. Chris Rehn recalls, 'We started as a cottage industry and it wasn't until later that we grew to become a much larger organisation'.

The day to day administrative tasks and politics of running the centre had previously been a juggling act for Bill, while he maintained a full surgical load. Alex commented in a speech she gave at a CICADA function that it was a relief for herself and Bill 'when into our lives came young Christopher Rehn, who arrived with such enthusiasm and is another one who loves and lives for the job'.

For the staff Christmas lunch in December, it was only a short walk down Punt Road to the Banjo Paterson restaurant, where Bill and Bob had celebrated their fiftieth birthdays. In the New Year, about twenty staff from both the children's and adults' implant programs drove up to Bill and Alex's holiday house at Diamond Beach for the first of many strategic planning weekends. Chris says that Alex did most of the 'heavy lifting' during this weekend, with regards to organisation and catering. She always took care of not only Bill, but all his staff.

Chris arranged for a paid facilitator to lead workshops, which tackled questions such as: 'How we can be everything our clients need us to be?' In the early years of the two cochlear implant programs, services needed to be provided in the city, but there was now a fair-sized cohort of children who lived in country towns. Chris suggested that the team put some computers in the back of his car and drive two hours north of Sydney to Newcastle to do the mapping sessions on some local children. Everyone liked this idea and the proposed visit would signal the beginning of their 'outreach service'.

The reward for the hard work during the strategic planning weekend were the festivities on the Saturday evening. Bill asked his tenants at Diamond Beach, Peter and Jackie, to take his staff out on a boat trip, where they had drinks and 'knickknacks', as Bill called the finger food, before staying the night at some holiday cabins near his holiday house.

Diamond Beach is a pristine 6-kilometre stretch of white sand, where Bill likes to unwind and go fishing with his friend Mike Cook, who, Chris notes, 'has a different take on life to Prof'. The day Mike, an ex-policeman, walked across the road and issued an invitation for Bill to 'go fishing' was the beginning of a lasting friendship and a great fishing partnership. Some holidays they caught so many fish that Mike had to walk up and down the street with a bucket giving them away to the neighbours.

* * *

Only two months after the strategic planning meeting, Bill was a session organiser for the 16th International Federation of Oto-rhino-laryngology Societies (IFOS) World Congress. Among the delegates present at the opening ceremony at the Sydney Opera House in March 1997 were Bill's UK friends David Moffat, Richard Ramsden and Jonathan Hazell. After the conference, Bill drove these three friends and a German colleague up to Diamond Beach.

On a trip into the nearest large town of Forster, Bill thought Richard Ramsden might like to spend his money in a two-dollar shop called Fair Dinkum Bargains. Ramsden described it as 'a scruffy shop that sold the most ghastly things'. However, they did purchase a brightly coloured gnome, which broke after much 'tomfoolery' back at the beach house. From then on, gnomes made regular appearances at conferences attended by Richard and Bill.

Richard told Bill a sad story about some parents who had brought their seven-year-old son to him for a cochlear implant. The parents said, 'We've been asking our doctor since he was two, "Is he old enough yet?" and the doctor kept saying, "No, not yet."' Bill says, 'Unfortunately, they had missed the critical period.'

Bill considered the ideal age for an infant to have a cochlear implant to be around nine months, because at that point they still have spontaneous babbling. Bill was quoted in a radio interview as saying, 'Babbling stops at that stage if the child is deaf. Everyone thinks this concept is too bold, but I am sure that it can be achieved.' If the auditory areas of the brain are not stimulated during this critical period of birth to nine months, Bill says that the brain will lose its ability to attach meaning to sound by stimulating the relevant 'association areas' of the brain. He was chuckling as he explained to Margaret Throsby during this radio interview, 'So for instance when my son hears "mother" it goes to the association area of his brain that says, "money", "car", "food" – whatever he associates with his mother.'[2]

Even before Jack McLeod was born, his parents were aware that there might be a problem with his hearing, because his mother Carol had contracted rubella during the first trimester of her pregnancy. As a newborn, Jack made no reaction at all when his parents clanged saucepans and took him to loud parties. On the day of his pre-implant assessment, Bill told Jack's parents to come back in a couple of months. Rob McLeod implored Bill to reconsider, saying, 'Look, you've implanted an infant at fourteen months of age – why not Jack at eleven months?'

After applying for permission from the Ethics Committee at the Children's Hospital at Westmead, Bill operated on Jack McLeod when he was twelve months old. Bill believes Jack then replaced Sally Wiltshire-Bridle as the youngest congenitally deaf child in the world to receive the Nucleus device. This prompted an invitation for Bill to appear on *Midday with Kerri-Anne*, hosted by Kerri-Anne Kennerley, along with Jack, his parents and an adult cochlear implant recipient, Steve Pascoe. Kerri-Anne told the studio audience that 'Recently the cochlear implant centre in New South Wales has been working miracles for the deaf'. She then said, 'Well, Professor ... how does it work?'[3] Bill explained how sound is heard while pointing to various components of a cochlear implant which were in a briefcase he had placed on a low coffee table.

Meanwhile, Jack was charming the studio audience, which included Alex Gibson and Chris Rehn, by crawling right up to the television cameras and peering into the lens. Then the briefcase caught Jack's eye and he crawled over to the coffee table. Bill recalls there being a collective sigh of relief from the audience when he managed to extricate Jack's arm just before the lid of the briefcase snapped shut.

Kerri-Anne then turned her attention to 43-year-old Steve Pascoe, who suffers from hereditary deafness. While other members of his family had gone deaf in their twenties, Steve said that the onset of his deafness had started much earlier. 'It was really incredibly devastating socially – going out with my friends – it was as if I had changed and they didn't accept me any more,' Steve told Kerri-Anne.

About nine months before the show, Bill had implanted Steve with one of the new Nucleus 24 implants (the CI24M) as part of a Clinical Research Centre trial. This latest offering from Cochlear, which Bill had also used for Jack McLeod's operation, had more rapid signal processing and two additional electrodes, which the surgeon did not place inside the cochlea, but reduced the energy needed for stimulation.

Even though Bill had been assisted from time to time by other surgeons including Barry Scrivener, Henley Harrison and Ted Beckenham, he had been the sole surgeon in the cochlear implant program for the previous thirteen years. In 1997, Cathy Birman joined Bill as a second surgeon working 'on a sessional basis', which involved having a portion of her operating sessions at a public hospital while maintaining her own private ENT practice.

The same year Bill purchased his own consulting rooms very near to RPA in a new development in Newtown called the Chancellory, on the corner of Missenden Road and Carillon Avenue. The foundation staff members for these private rooms were his wife Alex as the practice manager, Cathy Ball, who assisted with the electrophysiological testing, and Rose Ferris, who had come to work for Bill as a receptionist when Barry Scrivener retired. Scrivener died a few years later at the age of seventy-three and it made Bill ponder the question, 'Why do the people who are truly great have to be struck down?'

The first of Bill's fellows to be funded by the Graham Fraser Foundation, Tim Mitchell, was nearing the end of his six months of training. He helped Bill to carry his microscope and books across the road from the RPA Medical Centre, where Bill had previously seen his private patients, to these new rooms. All of the fellows conducted a study while they were in Australia. Tim's study compared the performance of children in the cochlear implant program who had congenital deafness with that of children who had acquired deafness.[4] The staff at the centre had noticed that it was reasonably common for the congenitally deaf group to have additional health concerns.

When the children's cochlear implant program was still located in Naremburn, Bill had performed a cochlear implant operation on a preschool-aged girl named Jessica, who suffered from Alport Syndrome, a rare condition affecting her kidneys and hearing. Maree Rennie, the aural habilitationist who had worked with Jessica after her implant, visited her not long before she died at the Children's Hospital at Randwick. Maree delivered the eulogy at Jessica's funeral, because she knew that Bill had endured the loss of a child of a similar age and would find this request from her parents incredibly difficult. The theme from *The Lion King* was Jessica's favourite and her parents gave Maree their daughter's toy lion, Simba, to take back to the centre for the other children with cochlear implants. This was a profoundly sad time for Bill and his team, which made them even more aware of the need for deaf children with complex needs to be able to communicate with their parents and receive comfort from them.

* * *

The cascade of just over one-hundred brand-new townhouses in Bill and Alex's complex on the Balmain peninsula overlooks a residents' marina, so Bill sold his trailer boat and bought an 8-metre cruiser. Some Danish neighbours owned a miniature schnauzer called Wolfie, who soon became their semi-permanent house guest. Bill says that when he and Alex decided to buy a female puppy of the same breed, 'Wolfie was a bit disdaining of Lilly at first, but later they became the best of friends'. One of the many pluses of Bill and Alex's new townhouse was its proximity to the city as well as to RPA, his office at the university and the Old Gladesville Hospital.

Jennie Brand-Miller began her position as a lecturer in nutrition at the University of Sydney at twenty-six, when her hearing was already deteriorating. She spent the next two decades battling to gain acceptance for the glycaemic index (GI), which measures the effect of foods on blood glucose. Chris Rehn thought that Jennie's journey was in many ways similar to that of his boss: 'Jennie fought the battle for GI, which is now one of the benchmarks of human nutrition. Prof fought for kids to have the cochlear implant. You know you're on to something great when people want to bring you down.'

By the time she was forty-six, Jennie was seriously considering retiring as a lecturer. She describes 'living under a black cloud', because she was finding it difficult to hear and answer the questions of her university students, despite wearing two high-powered hearing aids.[5] Jennie felt very fortunate to reside in the same city as Bill, who she considers to be one of the leading cochlear implant surgeons in the world. After her switch-on, Jennie walked out of Monica Bray's office into the grassy courtyard at Gladesville. She could hear birds twittering and said to herself, 'God! It's like I'm in an aviary'.

Even though Jennie had her pre-implant assessment at RPA, her post-implant appointments took place at Gladesville. This was after Bill had gained permission to have the children's and adults' programs located on the same site. Monica recalls that she and Denyse Rockey 'moved out of the dungeon at RPA Hospital and into the sunlight at Gladesville'. Monica and Denyse, who were still officially part of the RPA adult cochlear implant program, liked to wear white doctor's coats and it took Chris Rehn quite a while to convince them that they no longer needed to wear them.

The dungeon at RPA had never been the kind of place to host seminars so Monica was excited about having a conference room where her professional colleagues could be brought up to date on cochlear implants and become less sceptical about the technology. The day Bill stood in the middle of the conference room with Chris, admiring the fresh paintwork and new carpet, Alex turned up with their puppy Lilly, who christened the new carpet with 'a sprinkle of wee' – much to the disgust of the neat and orderly Chris.

Bill knew one of the audiologists who attended seminars in this new conference room at Gladesville, Professor Philip Newall, because they had attended audiology conferences together in the United Kingdom. Newall has retained his Manchester accent and he recalls Bill joking with him one day about how he sounded like Wallace from the *Wallace and Gromit* cartoons.

In 1980, Newall was appointed as the first full-time lecturer in audiology at Macquarie University, which subsequently gained a strong reputation for its graduate courses in this discipline. Bill became an honorary lecturer for the audiology students and also donated his services as the clinical director of the audiology clinic in the School of English, Linguistics and Media, where audiologists-in-training could be supervised while they conducted sessions with patients. Newall comments that this clinic was a critical step in the development of the Macquarie audiology program.

Sixty-seven-year old Roma Wood attended the audiology clinic at Macquarie University at the suggestion of one of her colleagues from Better Hearing Australia (BHA). Roma's deafness began in childhood and she didn't think that hearing again was a possibility until she was referred to Bill, who gave her the 'gentle encouragement' she needed to agree to a cochlear implant. For Roma, who has for many years provided lip-reading and hearing loss management classes at BHA, the teacher became the taught. Her audiologist Monica Bray passed the tissue box and said 'Keep going' when Roma shed tears of frustration. However, not long after her switch-on, Roma heard a new sound near the back door of her home and realised it was the tweeting of her canary.

Monica says Bill is known for taking a complete medical history of his patients, rather than only asking about their ears. She recalls that one person told him that their sense of smell was altered and his enquiries revealed a tumour on their olfactory nerve. It was a persistent cough that triggered alarm bells for Bill in 53-year-old Libby Harricks, who referred to herself as 'the deaf pharmacist'. During her pre-implant assessment, Libby mentioned to Bill, 'I have this little cough that won't go away'. Bill noticed the previous occurrence of breast cancer in her clinical notes and ordered a chest X-ray, which revealed multiple metastases.

'She was so young. Breast cancer is the sword of Damocles for a woman, like prostate cancer is for a man. Libby thought she was clear of the cancer, but you never know when it's going to come back,' says Bill, who had treated Libby for many years before she fell ill and subsequently died. 'In her role as the first president of the government's peak body for hearing, the Deafness Forum, Libby was a calming influence and helped a lot with the politics.'

Many close associates were concerned about Bill when they saw him arrive at Libby's funeral with a bandage wound around his partially shaved head. He had developed headaches after banging his head on a theatre light, and presented himself to Accident and Emergency for a CT scan. Bill remembers the doctor and technician looking 'grim-faced' when they told him he had a subdural haematoma, which required an operation to drill drainage holes in his skull. Bill discovered that he had a bleeding tendency, which he shares with Bob and has passed on to his children, 'much to their joy,' he adds wryly.

On Saturday mornings, Bill and Alex sometimes stroll through the farmers' markets at Rozelle Public School on the Balmain peninsula to buy fresh produce and free-range eggs. Bill was in a cheeky mood the weekend he put a note into each of his neighbours' letterboxes, saying: 'Alex and I would like to keep some chickens on our balcony. If you have any objections, let us know by the 1st of April.' They received one note back straight away from the neighbours in the townhouse directly opposite, who said, 'If you are going to keep chickens, we should be able to keep pigs. Then we can have eggs and bacon.' They clearly got the joke, but not so an Italian neighbour who knocked on their front door with the note clenched tightly in his fist. Bill said, 'Look, we can share the eggs with you if you like'. The neighbour refused to be bribed, saying, 'I don't want any of that'. Bill then broke into a smile and asked him, 'What date is it today, Mimo?'

It was too far for Bill to drive to Berowra Rotary from Balmain so he joined the Haberfield Rotary Club at the recommendation of a social contact, Glenn Wran. Bill found support for his implant programs at his new Rotary Club and also from Wran, who agreed to take on the role of chairman of the EAR Foundation after Bert Hely's departure. Glenn introduced the proceedings at an evening dinner function held in a marquee in the courtyard of the Old Gladesville Hospital to celebrate the centre's 500th cochlear implant surgery. He then handed the microphone to Adam Spencer from radio station Triple J for the first of his many appearances as master of ceremonies for the centre's fundraisers.

The next day an article about the event appeared in a local newspaper, the *Weekly Times*, surrounded by advertisements from businesses in the area and several members of parliament congratulating Bill and the members of his team on reaching this milestone.[6] They were now the second-largest cochlear implant program worldwide. The largest program was established in Hannover by Ernst Lehnhardt, who, like Bill, started implanting patients with the Nucleus device in August 1984 and was another pioneer of this branch of surgery.[7]

The first time Margaret Throsby invited Bill to appear on her hour-long drive-time radio program on ABC Classic FM, he spoke about establishing his cochlear implant program in New South Wales and the optimal age to perform the operation on babies. In between his musical choices, Bill also told Margaret the story of an 86-year-old man who previously would disappear to his room whenever visitors appeared, but, after his cochlear implant, made a point of coming out and dominating the conversation. Margaret asked Bill, 'So it's never too late?' and Bill replied, 'No way!'[8]

A 76-year-old artist named Allan Waite would later write in a tribute to his surgeon that he had been preparing to resign as the leader of a group of artists known as the 'Plein Air Painters' when 'along came the Prof with his bag of tricks and bestowed on me such a wonderful renaissance'. On the day of his surgery, Allan took a photo of Bill in his green theatre garb which he later used to paint his portrait. Allan was a talented war and landscape artist and his portrait of Bill still hangs on a wall of the cochlear implant centre in Gladesville.

When the volunteer support group CICADA was approached by an equivalent patient group from Japan requesting a visit, Bill as the chairman of the Australian group felt apprehensive for a couple of reasons. Most of the Japanese group spoke little English and the Australians spoke no Japanese. The only exceptions were an Australian implant recipient named Kazuko Scott and her husband Mal, who she had met when he was involved in peace-keeping efforts as an Australian soldier in Hiroshima. Bill's other concern was the number of Australian war veterans among the implantees who would be attending the wine and cheese evening at the Cochlear offices. Bill's fears turned out to be unfounded and he wrote in his editorial for a new national newsletter of CICADA groups across Australia, 'The common bond of deafness and being a user of a cochlear implant seemed to overcome all barriers. After twenty minutes it would have seemed to any casual spectator that everyone was conversing with a familiar friend.' A few of the Japanese ladies were wearing kimonos and there was some discussion about the best place to put their speech processors. Bill remembers Shirley Hanke pointing down her top and saying, 'I keep my processor between my boobs', which produced bursts of giggles all round.

Shirley Hanke had been inspired to write a book, *The Story of CICADA*, after a visit to the Powerhouse Museum in Sydney, where she discovered that a display of early cochlear implant technology had been removed. This display had included an oval glass-topped table with prototype implants and wire headbands, above which there had been a plaque listing the first group of implant recipients. Shirley was concerned that their efforts would be forgotten so she collected the stories of thirty-four early cochlear implant recipients in New South Wales. Bill wrote in the preface to her book, 'The successes and disappointments of cochlear implants only became evident because of their experiences'.[9] In September 2000, Shirley was very pleased when Catherine Livingstone, the CEO of Cochlear, wrote the message which appeared on the front inside cover of her book.

* * *

For Judy Cassell, memories of her cochlear implant operation, when she was fifty-three, are entwined with the Sydney Olympics of 2000. The previous year she had attended the opening of the Olympic stadium with her husband Peter, and recalls feeling 'frightened and overwhelmed' by the crowds because she had recently lost the remainder of her hearing. Bill was able to perform her cochlear implant operation during the school holidays, so Judy could return the next term to her job as a high school textile and design teacher.

In the lead-up to Christmas each year, Bill and several staff members were invited to a graduation ceremony for school-aged children who were departing the Shepherd Centre. The director, Bruce Shepherd, approached Bill to suggest that the Shepherd Centre take over the cochlear implants for children with deafness as their single disability. This would have left Bill and his team with the adults and children with multiple disabilities. Bill remembers Bruce Shepherd becoming quite upset when his offer was rejected. However, Bill firmly believed that it was preferable all for the children referred to his program to be implanted by the one centre.

Christmas is always a busy time for Bill and Alex, spending time with their family, which by now included three grandsons: Jack, Sam and a new baby, Joe. Laura's family had moved to Port Macquarie, where Stephen works at the hospital as a consultant oncologist. It takes Bill and Alex an hour to drive from Diamond Beach to the Begbies' home, overlooking the lighthouse at Tacking Point. Bill usually makes a model of a house to put in the middle of the table on Christmas day, as his father had once done. But one year, when Laura and Stephen hosted the Gibson family Christmas lunch, Bill used cardboard tubing to make a model of a lighthouse and placed little presents inside.

Chris Rehn asked Amy, one of the audiologists at Gladesville (and his future wife), if she would drive with him up to Diamond Beach. He had woken during the night with an 'Aha' moment and wanted to tell Bill his good idea in person. On the way up, Chris and Amy discussed the fact that the kids were located upstairs in their wing of the Old Gladesville Hospital with their own waiting room, while the adults were downstairs with their own waiting room. On their arrival, Chris posed the inevitable question: 'Prof, why don't we combine the children's and adults' implant programs?'

Just as it had been difficult to prise the white doctor's coats from the backs of the adult audiologists, Monica Bray and Denyse Rockey,

Bill now had to convince them to be part of a combined cochlear implant program. 'They thought they'd be swallowed alive, but they didn't realise that one day there would be far more adults than children.' The year 2001 marked the beginning of the not-for-profit charity: the Sydney Cochlear Implant Centre (SCIC). An SCIC board was formed and a stylised swirl, representing the spirals inside the cochlea, replaced Sidney the snail as the centre's logo.

The same year, Bill performed a cochlear implant operation on a 75-year-old man, the Reverend Burn Reeve, who said to him, 'Do you realise you have also implanted my great-granddaughter Alicia, from the [NSW] town of Parkes?' Bill told Reverend Reeve, 'This is history', because their family epitomised the life-long service that he and Chris hoped to create with the SCIC.

The combined adults' and children's cochlear implant program had clients ranging in age from their late eighties down to babies such as five-month-old Harry, who had Pendred Syndrome – a genetic disorder that leads to hearing loss and decreased thyroid function. When the SCIC habilitation staff analysed their database of children who had received cochlear implants in the program, approximately 20 per cent had a disability in addition to their hearing loss.[10]

Historically, children who were deaf and had additional disabilities such as intellectual challenges, autism or cerebral palsy might not have been offered hearing aids or glasses. Maree Rennie says that these children were initially also not considered as candidates for cochlear implants and some clinics still take this position. 'Many children were placed in institutions after their parents were given the bad news: the train will leave but never arrive at the station.' The SCIC did not have the facilities or funds to provide the intensive therapy these children required, but inspiration for a new home-like centre came from a special little girl, Matilda Rose, whose parents were determined to secure a bright and happy future for her.

CHAPTER 13

The best use of the money

We knew there would be some children who would attend mainstream schools and maybe even university, and others who would continue to need a more specialised educational setting, but you don't know the outcome for an individual child until you try.

Maree Rennie, coordinator,
RIDBC Matilda Rose Centre

Matilda Rose Carnegie's parents brought her to Bill for an assessment for a cochlear implant when she was three months old. She had her cochlear implant operation six months later and the aural habilitationist, Maree Rennie, became her case manager. In addition to her profound deafness, Matilda had disabilities including mild cerebral palsy and macrodactyly of her right foot.

Unfortunately, Matilda was overwhelmed by the auditory information she was receiving from her cochlear implant, which made habilitation sessions and social interactions stressful for both her and her parents, Tanya and Mark Carnegie. In 2000, when Matilda was three, she was refused entry to preschool because of her poor communication skills and repetitive behaviour, which included rocking and humming. The Carnegies wanted someone to work one-on-one with their daughter and engaged the services of Maree Rennie, who has a master's degree in education from Boston in working with children with deafness, blindness and multiple disabilities. She also has a reputation as being the equivalent of a 'horse whisperer' for her ability to soothe and relate to a child who feels frustrated by his or her disabilities.

From the success of these sessions, and through extensive consultations with experts in the field of deaf and blind children such as Judy Simser, Jan van Dijk and Jan North, came the idea of creating a new centre, where teachers could provide specialised intensive therapy for children aged two to six, to help them reach their full potential. Tanya and Mark established the Carnegie Foundation in 2000, which purchased a cottage next to their own historic home, Ellsmore, in Sydney's eastern suburbs. The Carnegies collaborated with Bill and the CEO of the SCIC, Chris Rehn, to establish a centre in this cottage in 2001, which they named the Matilda Rose Early Intervention Centre. Tanya Nelson Carnegie became the founding director and two of the SCIC staff, Maree Rennie and Terry Meskin, were the founding teachers.

The first year there was a small class of only five deaf children, including Matilda Rose. The teachers focused not only on their ears but their minds and bodies. The former president of Cochlear Asia Pacific (2004–2014), Mark Salmon, says that some people might ask, 'Is that the best use of the money?' He says that Bill would tell them, 'Of course it's worth it. You're making a huge difference to those children's future lives.'

Just as he had for his mother in 1984, Bill found himself once again returning to England to see a parent in declining health. This time, in 2001, after playing a key role in establishing a program for deaf children with additional disabilities, he was visiting his father, who had oesophageal cancer.

Bill picked up a hire car at Heathrow Airport and drove the four hours down to Devon, but when he arrived at the Dawlish Cottage Hospital, the more senior of the two nurses took him into a little side room and said, 'You're too late … Your father died two hours ago.' The next day Eleanor told him about his father's last days and soon afterwards, Kathy arrived from Canada and Bob from Australia. Instead of organising a ninetieth birthday celebration for their father, the four Gibson siblings arranged his funeral, which included blue flowers – in lieu of the out-of-season cornflowers – in their buttonholes and draped over his coffin.

In his eulogy at St Gregory's in Dawlish, Bill said: 'It is hard to say goodbye to Dad, or as my brother and I used to say "our father".' He later showed the typed sheet of words to Laura, who said, 'Were you able to say all that, Dad?' and he replied, 'Only just; my voice got a bit trembly'. Bill wrote an obituary for the Epsom College Journal. With the assistance of his brother-in-law from Northampton, Bill wrote a second obituary for the *British Medical Journal*[1] – the journal where Richard Marshall had encouraged him to publish his first clinical paper.

* * *

Early in Bill's medical career, two of the main causes of deafness acquired *in utero* were rubella and Rhesus incompatibility, but these cases are now quite rare. A more recent cause of deafness in newborns is prematurity, which increases the risk of deafness from one in 1000 live births to one in one hundred – in other words, by a factor of ten.[2]

Zoe Dunn was born at twenty-nine weeks and the hospital staff reassured her parents, saying, 'You don't need to worry about her hearing. Zoe passed the otoacoustic emissions [OAE] test.' Around nine months Zoe was not meeting her physical milestones and was diagnosed with cerebral palsy. Then, at around eighteen months, an auditory brainstem response test revealed what her mother, Catherine, had suspected for some time. She says, 'Zoe's audiogram was right down low where people can't even hear jet engines and rock bands. The original OAE test was a false positive result.' During Zoe's assessment for a cochlear implant, Catherine could tell they were in good hands because Bill was 'so warm and kind in his approach'.

Catherine also had a feeling that the Matilda Rose Centre was the right place for her daughter. When she was told there were no places for the next preschool year, Maree asked her co-director Tanya if she could accept another child, and Tanya agreed. A couple of years later Zoe's smiling face featured on the front of a brochure for the centre.

Through the Carnegie Foundation, Tanya and Mark poured what Maree believes to be millions of dollars into this centre in running costs, salaries for teachers and therapists, as well as professional training. Maree stated, 'They'd never let people know what they've done, but they've given hope to so many people'.[3] Catherine and James Dunn remember the day Bill thanked the Carnegies for all their assistance with the 'Mary Rose Centre' and thought he must have mistakenly referred to Henry VIII's Tudor flagship. After a few awkward moments, Bill corrected his slip and the audience broke into enthusiastic applause.

The Matilda Rose Centre was one of the places Bill brought his Graham Fraser fellows during their six-month stay in Sydney. During the first half of 2002, this was Peter Rea (whose name coincidentally is the same as Bill's middle names). Rea was able to follow the progress of several children from diagnosis to cochlear implant operation and wrote in his Fellowship report, 'I know of no comparable period of training available anywhere in the world'.[4]

Peter Rea also assisted Bill with some important research to find a suitable screening test for deaf babies. Bill recalls that the NSW Minister for Health, Craig Knowles, was keen to pursue this testing, because it made good financial sense. 'You save quite a lot of money in the long run,' says Bill, 'because deaf children who receive cochlear implants at an early age usually don't need to attend special schools.' A NSW Department of Education and Training Annual Report in 2000 estimated the cost of teacher's aides, special education services and special schools for one deaf child to be $118 000 per year, which the report stated was five times the cost of mainstream education.

In 2001 Bill was invited to join the Universal Newborn Hearing Screening Reference Group, to explore options for the most suitable hearing test for newborns.[5] Some Australian states, including Victoria and Western Australia, advocated the OAE test. Bill told Craig Knowles and the co-members of this reference group that this test was unsuitable, because it produces false positive and false negative results. The research he conducted with his fellow Peter Rea revealed that nearly half of all deaf babies born under thirty-six weeks' gestation pass the test (a false positive result).[6] This is because the OAE test picks up emissions from 'outer hair cells', which cannot send sound messages along the hearing nerve to the brain. Disturbingly, some children with normal hearing also fail the test (a false negative result), so in Bill's opinion it was 'not safe'.

Members of the reference group agreed unanimously with Bill's suggestion of using the automated auditory brain stem response (AABR) test instead of the OAE test. Bill believes it was due to the hard work of the group's chair, Elizabeth Murphy, that New South Wales became one of the first places in the world to introduce Statewide Infant Screening – Hearing (SWISH), using only AABR on babies. Within hours of their birth, babies are tested via a painless procedure, and those who don't pass the test are referred for a detailed audiological assessment.

Fifteen months after the commencement of SWISH, in December 2002, Bill became a member of the NSW Ministerial Committee on Hearing, formed to discuss the SWISH program, diagnostic audiology services in area health and cochlear implant programs in New South Wales.[7] For the next decade Bill attended these bi-monthly meetings of several hours' duration in North Sydney, which were initially chaired by the NSW Health Minister, Peter Anderson, and then by Professor Jennie Brand-Miller. It was a big commitment for someone like Bill, who already had a heavy surgical and travel load.

When Bill attended the Seventh International Cochlear Implant Conference in Manchester in 2002, protestors against the use of cochlear implants in hearing-impaired children paraded coffins outside the convention centre, and delegates had to be ushered in via a side door. Bill contributed a lighter note to the plenary session when he presented a gnome in bubble wrap to his friend Richard Ramsden, the conference organiser, who unwrapped it on stage and held it up for the delegates to see.

It transpired that each of the nine or so coffins paraded outside the convention centre represented a child who had died from meningitis as a complication of a cochlear implant operation. An investigation revealed that the common denominator in the deaths, which occurred at centres around the world, including several cases in Spain, was the use of the US-designed Advanced Bionics (AB) 'positioner', which was used to push the electrode array closer to the modiolus, in the centre of the cochlea. It was shown that this positioner allowed micro-organisms to enter the inner ear via a small gap, and the AB device which included this positioner was withdrawn from the market.

Bill wrote a 'safety alert' to reassure the families of the SCIC that there were no documented cases of meningitis resulting from a cochlear implant operation in Sydney, or in fact anywhere in Australia. The SCIC had strict safety protocols to prevent infections, which involved quarantining the child for one week before and two weeks after their surgery. During this time, no play dates or classes in centres with other children were permitted.

* * *

Bill's next fellow, Jaydip Ray, said the Gibsons' hospitality started the first day his family moved into their rental accommodation at Balmoral Beach. Alex provided a car trailer containing many of the household goods they would need, ranging from cots to pots and pans. When Ray returned to University College Hospital, he wrote a report for the trustees of the Graham Fraser Foundation in which he summarised his six months in Australia as being an abundance of 'Sun, sea, sand, surf and SURGERY'.[8] Bill offered what was principally a surgical Fellowship, which some fellows referred to as 'the otology finishing school' or 'the apprenticeship'. Although Bill does remember hosting one Irish fellow, Brendan Conlon, who was 'very keen on writing papers, but was difficult to coax into the operating theatres'.

Most of the UK fellows would comment on the strong emphasis the SCIC placed on fundraising, which is unusual in their home country, where the NHS decides who can have an implant. Fundraising allowed Bill and his centre manager Chris Rehn to allocate cochlear implants and habilitation to approximately one-hundred public patients from their waiting lists, including the twenty-two implants per year paid for by the NSW government.

The demand for outreach services was growing rapidly, with SCIC staff making regular visits to fifteen locations around New

South Wales, in towns as far away as Tamworth, Lismore and Wagga Wagga. Demand for services was particularly strong in Newcastle, two hours north of Sydney, and one of Bill's implant recipients, Max Lindsay, organised all kinds of fundraisers, including 'chook raffles', to encourage the establishment of a centre in his home city. When a permanent branch in Newcastle seemed likely, Chris and Bill both smiled and shook their heads as they remarked to each other: 'Why did we put Sydney in our name?'

The SCIC staff saw adult outreach clients at the country offices of the Commonwealth government agency Australian Hearing, while children were seen at several of the Royal Institute for Deaf and Blind Children (RIDBC) schools. Bill also referred children with cochlear implants from the SCIC to these RIDBC schools if they needed special education, so the year 2003 will be remembered as the beginning of a two-way collaboration between these two not-for-profit organisations. During the six years they had worked together, Chris developed a strong rapport with Bill and had also come to know his family well. This includes Bill's son Hugh, who is a similar age to Chris.

When Hugh announced his engagement to Catherine Purcell, he told his family that it was possible for them to be married in the Naval Chapel at Garden Island in Sydney Harbour because her father is a retired rear admiral. Until Hugh's marriage, Bill had been the custodian of the Gibson family grandfather clock, which had come across from England in a sea container after the death of his father. John wanted it to be passed down the Gibson line to Hugh, his only grandson. Bill and Alex had the clock restored and delivered to Hugh and Cate's home in the inner west of Sydney, not far from where they live on the Balmain peninsula.

When another townhouse in their complex came up for sale, Bill and Alex were quick to act. Their new townhouse had the advantage of being on the water's edge and a stroll of only 50 metres away from the marina, where Bill moored his latest cruising motor boat, *Mad Wax*. There was even a small garden, accessed from the lower level, for their schnauzer Lilly to 'do her business'.

Bill is still a keen jogger, but he no longer feels up to competing in the annual 14-kilometre City2Surf, which became a fundraiser on the SCIC calendar each August. The group of staff and patients, who ran in coordinating T-shirts, called themselves 'Team Farrell', because forming the team was the idea of the Farrell family, whose wheelchair-bound sons Bradley and Thomas both suffered from a rare genetic condition called Arts Syndrome.[9] The Farrells pushed their sons around the course with the assistance of staff and teachers from both the SCIC and the Matilda Rose Centre.

Bill made visits to this centre as often as he could, to see how the children were progressing, and Maree Rennie laughs as she recalls him sticking his head out from the door of the staff 'loo' to shout his ideas out to her. He encouraged the teachers to publish their research on attachment theory and social connection. Children with complex needs often have insecure attachment due to anxiety and stress, which makes it more difficult for them to identify and process auditory stimuli.[10] The staff aim to optimise the connection between the children and their family or significant others, to help them form loving relationships. They also instil in the children a strong belief in themselves and the importance of reaching for the highest of their abilities.

The centre in Bronte was set up to have a family-like atmosphere where parents were welcome. Catherine and James Dunn have a photo of Zoe lying on the floor of the centre twiddling the dials of an electronic musical toy, and they have written in the speech bubble above it, 'I can hear that sound'. Maree Rennie and Terry Meskin included everyday activities in their curriculum, such as cooking and learning how to wash hands. A couple of years after the centre was established, the Carnegies provided additional funding for an increased number of students and professional staff, including an occupational therapist and a physiotherapist.

The staff of the SCIC at Gladesville viewed the children and activities of the Matilda Rose Centre in Bronte as a special extension of their own work. Updates on the centre appeared in the SCIC newsletters and Maree Rennie was invited to speak for the seminar series held in the SCIC conference room.

* * *

The regular Tuesday evening seminars at the SCIC feature an invited speaker and attract continuing education points for the audiologists who attend. The final seminar of the year includes inspirational talks by cochlear implant recipients and festive treats afterwards, provided by a sponsor. As the director of the centre, Bill usually began his opening address with: 'I always knew when spring was approaching in England, because of the call of the cuckoo bird. I know when Christmas is approaching here in Australia, because it is time to attend, "Where are they now?"'

One of the talks at the December 2004 seminar was given by a young woman, Xanthe McLean, whose hearing started to deteriorate from the age of four. Despite having severe to profound hearing loss during her high school years, Xanthe scored just over ninety-five from a possible one hundred in the NSW Higher School Certificate. However, this A-grade student reached her tipping point in the decision to go ahead with a cochlear implant when she failed the first clinical placement in her physiotherapy degree. She had difficulty communicating with her patients on the wards and this was seen as a safety issue. Xanthe told the seminar audience that her cochlear implant had allowed her to work in her 'dream career'. During informal discussions with Bill, Xanthe says that he treats her like a professional colleague, and one of their points of connection is that his daughter Laura is also a physiotherapist.

It was the new IT manager at the SCIC, Steve Pascoe, who had set up the audiovisual equipment for this seminar. When Bill performed cochlear implant surgery on Steve in 1997, he was working in a senior IT and project management role for the Defence Force. His new role involved setting up the necessary infrastructure across multiple sites for the SCIC to function effectively as a growing service. When the SCIC conducted a study of single-implant recipients who had decided to have a second implant, Steve Pascoe enrolled as a research participant. One of the coordinators of the bilateral project was the diagnostic and research audiologist Kirsty Gardner-Berry, who, like Steve, had recently joined the SCIC team. Steve and Kirsty would later work together on a project to develop remote mapping services for the SCIC and would also become life partners.

Bill initially erred on the side of caution with the trend towards bilateral implantation, particularly in children, as the feeling had been that one ear should be 'saved' in case of future treatments and improved technology. But soon the benefits of hearing from two ears instead of one – such as more directional hearing – would lead to more people requesting a second cochlear implant. One of Bill's very early implant recipients, Alan Jones, decided to have a second implant in 1999 because he wanted to take advantage of the recently released behind-the-ear (BTE) speech processor. The BTE was a breakthrough for implant recipients, who no longer had the inconvenience of a body-worn speech processor, but Alan was also impressed with the improvements to the surgical experience. 'Oh, what a difference! Up and showered in eighteen hours, a small incision barely visible and nil loss of hair. The good professor had certainly got his act together over the last fourteen years.'[11]

Shirley Hanke was similarly impressed with the small incision when she had her second implant on 19 January 2004, nineteen years to the day since her first cochlear implant. Sue Walters was initially hesitant, preferring to stay with just her 'old standard', as she calls the device Bill implanted in 1984. It would be another year before she could be persuaded to have a second implant, by which time Cochlear had launched their 'Freedom' speech processor and matching cochlear implant, which utilised many more electrodes than Sue's older device. During her switch-on, Sue recalls that she ripped her Freedom speech processor off her head when the first sounds came through, because it felt like 'a high-speed train coming through a tunnel'. However, with the right programming, Sue became quite comfortable with her new speech processor and now prefers using it for telephone calls.

Bill says that it is very common for new bilateral recipients to experience a difficult first few weeks or even months as the other side of their brain adapts and forms new neural pathways. He tells people that the change is not nearly as dramatic after the second implant as it is after the first, and provides the analogy: 'It's like driving along and putting one headlight on and then putting on the other headlight'.

In the after-dinner speech Sue Walters gave on 13 August 2004 at the Gladesville RSL Club to mark the 20th anniversary of her first implant operation, she said that she had learnt to appreciate 'more of the little things in life', such as hearing the voices of her three children, who were now aged ten, eight and six. Two years before this dinner, Sue had started working at the SCIC as a clinical support officer, which involves troubleshooting for cochlear implant speech processors and accessories. She was speaking from the perspective of both a patient and a colleague when she said, '[Prof] has led the way in establishing the SCIC as a centre of excellence – the first of its kind in the world – and we're very proud of him'.

Many prominent people made an effort to attend Sue's anniversary dinner, including the new CEO of Cochlear, Chris

Roberts, and the former CEO of Nucleus, Paul Trainor. Trainor told a few people on the night that he had only agreed to commercialise Graeme Clark's prototype bionic ear on the condition that he transfer his 'best man' from Melbourne to Sydney to work at Nucleus. This was, of course, the engineer Jim Patrick, who moved to Sydney in 1981 and became the head of research for the Cochlear division of Nucleus. In 1984, Trainor acquired a second engineer from Clark's team, Peter Seligman, who had previously played a key role in reducing the size of the speech processor from a binocular-case-sized package that weighed about 7 kilograms to something wearable.

The project to produce the commercially viable Nucleus device succeeded because it combined what is sometimes referred to as the 'holy trinity' of university, industry and government. At a luncheon in 2004, held at the Australian Museum in Sydney, called 'Break the Silence', Bill and the other SCIC surgeon, Cathy Birman, sat at the head table with former Australian prime minister Malcolm Fraser, who told the audience that he had decided to take a chance on the cochlear implant technology and approve Commonwealth funding totalling over $4 million.

* * *

In the early years of his cochlear implant program, Bill would have found it difficult to believe that by 2004 they would have reached their 1000th implant surgery. This was performed by Cathy Birman on an eight-month-old baby girl, Ruby Loosemore. During a cele-bratory picnic held on a cricket oval within the grounds of the Old Gladesville Hospital, a photo was taken of Bill with Sue Walters and Cathy Birman, who is holding baby Ruby in her arms. There were brightly coloured marquees and guest appearances by two celebrities from the popular television soapie *Home and Away*, but the highlight of the day for Bill was an attempt at the world record for 'biggest gathering of cochlear implant recipients'. He wore a bright green outfit and is seated in the middle of the spiral-shaped crowd in the photo taken for the record attempt, which he recalls needed to be taken from a cherry-picker.

Events such as this picnic were organised by the SCIC's fundraising and development officer, Barbara Howard. Bill particularly enjoyed the dress-up events Barbara organised, and made an effort to look the part dressed as characters such as the Joker, in full face paint with a floppy hat. One of the attendees of a dress-up function called 'Arabian Nights – 1001 stories' was the director of the Renwick Centre at the RIDBC, Professor Greg Leigh, who Bill knew from the committee meetings of the Newborn Hearing Screening Reference Group. Professor Leigh attempted to strike up a conversation with Bob Gibson, who pointed to the other side of the marquee and said, 'If you want to speak to Bill, he's the one over there dressed like a sheik'. Bill was wearing dark sunglasses and a white caftan trimmed in electric blue, which he claims is 'very authentic' because it had been presented to him at an ENT conference in Saudi Arabia.

In his speech at this fundraiser, Bill mentioned that the ages of the implant recipients in their program now ranged from four-and-a-half months to ninety-four years. He joked that this could be interpreted as 'from basket to casket' or 'from birth to earth'. He has 'oodles' of variations on this expression, but his favourite is 'creation to cremation'.

The next person to mount the couple of steps up to the stage in the marquee was the nonagenarian implantee, Sylvia MacCormick, who Bill says is 'quite a character'. She shared the story of how she was deafened by the 'complications from a World War II bombing raid in London', where she was working as an ambulance driver. This led to severe hearing loss by the time she was in her forties, so she had missed hearing the voices of her extended family for fifty years.

Catherine and James Dunn attended the Arabian Nights fundraiser and hoped in the years ahead to be able to bring their two young daughters, Zoe and Phoebe, to such an inspirational event. They can remember Sylvia's speech and how much she enjoyed hearing the voices of her great-grandchildren. This remarkable 91-year-old told the audience that she hoped her cochlear implant would allow her to continue delivering Meals on Wheels to the 'old' people in the Sydney municipality of Mosman. When the Dunns looked around the crowded marquee, they noticed 'there wasn't a dry eye in the place'.

When Zoe Dunn turned six, she followed in the footsteps of Matilda Rose Carnegie to attend St Catherine's School for girls in Waverley, but she still came to the Matilda Rose Centre some afternoons after school. The combined approach of occupational therapy and physiotherapy utilised at the cottage helped Zoe learn to walk with a walking frame, despite her cerebral palsy. Her mother Catherine remembers the day Zoe walked across the room unaided at the age of seven and the staff were all cheering and crying at the same time. In the years ahead, Zoe would become a *Doctor Who* fan and receive awards at school for science, maths and diligence.

Bill is proud of all the children who have passed through the doors of the Matilda Rose Centre, including Zoe and Matilda, who had by now developed into a confident and accomplished girl of seven. When she was in Year 5 at St Catherine's, the Labour parliamentary secretary for the seat of Bennelong, Maxine McKew, read in parliament the speech Matilda made to her classmates, because she thought these words 'spoke volumes' about the exceptional future that lay ahead for this bright little girl and wanted them to be put on the public record:

> Imagine being deaf for a day? You know how it is
> when someone presses the mute button on the TV,
> but now instead imagine they pressed it on your life.

Imagine waking up and not hearing anything, not
even your alarm clock or the garbage trucks at 6 am.
Being deaf is like living in only part of the world, but
I don't have to live in only part of the world because
I have a cochlear implant, which lets me hear. What
it does is makes me hear really well when there is
just one person talking to me. However, in group
conversations it sounds like a hundred voices
speaking at once and it is overwhelming for me.
I am not asking for sympathy, instead just a bit of
consideration. But at the end of the day, just like
being tall, being deaf is part of what makes me
ME!![12]

The Matilda Rose Centre would soon expand into a second cottage on an adjoining block of land. The centre's co-directors, Maree Rennie and Tanya Nelson Carnegie, would also present their theories about social attachment and sensory integration at international conferences and their own annual workshop for professionals. Maree Rennie says that when she and Bill became involved in establishing the centre, their aim was to help this special cohort of children learn how to listen and be included in family and community life. 'We knew there would be some children who would attend mainstream schools and maybe even university and others who would continue to need a more specialised educational setting, but you don't know the outcome for an individual child until you try.'

CHAPTER 14

Dreams becoming a reality

Sufferers call it the 'dizzy terror'. More
than 50 000 Australians experience it.
The lives of millions are devastated by it,
baffling doctors around the world.

Menière's Research Fund[1]

Chrissy Boyce and her husband Johnny were the resident managers of the Mungo National Park in south-western New South Wales when she noticed that she could no longer hear the park's call signal. Her kids had to call out to her, 'Mum, someone is on radio 801!' A few years after returning to their home in the Sydney suburb of Mona Vale, Chrissy began experiencing nausea and light-headedness and became so 'wobbly' she was worried that neighbours would label her a heavy drinker. Chrissy was by now in her late forties and doctors told her 'It's the change of life' or 'It's all in your head'.

In the weeks leading up to her first appointment with Bill, Chrissy suffered her first frightening bout of giddiness and vomiting, which was so severe she couldn't even sit on a chair without falling off. Bill told Chrissy that most people, including doctors, underestimate the suffering caused by the attacks of vertigo in Menière's disease. He suggested an operation called a labyrinthectomy to remove the vestibular apparatus (balance organ) from her affected ear, and said, 'While I have your head open, I will pop in a cochlear implant'. When Chrissy had her operation on Remembrance Day in 1998, she was one of the first people in the world to have these two surgical procedures simultaneously.

After her operation, Chrissy described her hearing as 'great' but it took many months to regain her balance because her brain needed time to adjust to relying on the balance organ in her other ear. Chrissy will always have Menière's disease but her attacks of vertigo are now under control as long as she follows Bill's advice to keep her stress levels down and watch the level of salt in her diet.

Finding a cure for Menière's disease has been a long-held dream for Bill and he was excited to be acting in an advisory role for the NSW Menière's Support Group, which was raising funds for further research into this disorienting disease. In the meantime, Bill had a hierarchy of options ranging from 'reassurance' on the bottom rung of the ladder to 'cochlear implant' at the top, with many drug treatments and surgical procedures in between.[2]

In May 2005, at the launch of the Nucleus Freedom cochlear implant system, the CEO of Cochlear, Chris Roberts, said in his speech that the company had invested close to $100 million to produce their new-generation device and companion speech processor.[3] Sue Walters was one of the early recipients of the new technology and her audiologist at the SCIC, Monica Bray, said that if the wearable speech processor Sue received in 1984 was similar to viewing an Impressionist painting, by the mid-1990s it was like a colour television picture and now, with the Freedom, it was like a plasma screen. The name Freedom suited its cordless and splash-proof design.

The same year Cochlear released Freedom, several of Bill's patients became involved in a company initiative called the Cochlear Awareness Network (CAN), where they share their stories with community groups. Chrissy Boyce, who had previously described herself as 'a very reserved person', told Bill that 'the boost to her confidence after her cochlear implant was 80 per cent'. She was ready the day someone from CAN rang and asked, 'Chrissy, do you have a current passport? We need someone to give a presentation on the Freedom in Korea next week.'

Bilateral Freedom user and CAN advocate Faye Yarroll has spoken to 35 000 people and she is still going. Faye was in her mid-forties and working as an IT manager for Hewlett-Packard when she lost the remaining 12 per cent of her hearing in a case of codeine toxicity after injuring her back. Through in-depth interviewing, Monica Bray discovered ten more SCIC clients with similar clinical histories in the same calendar year. Bill provided the medical reviews for a study, which was the first to show a correlation between high doses of the over-the-counter pain reliever codeine – either alone or combined with other medications – and sudden hearing loss.[4]

In a few years' time Bill and Monica would both become recipients of the inaugural Cochlear Hearo Awards for 'delivering best patient outcomes' and Faye would be recognised for her tireless involvement with CAN in raising awareness about cochlear implants for deafened adults.[5] Through this network, Cochlear discovered what Bill and other members of the volunteer support group CICADA had known for a long time – that a story told by a cochlear implant recipient is far more inspiring than a marketing brochure.

* * *

Bill and Alex, in their role as patrons of CICADA, attended nearly all the Sunday barbecues held at the SCIC. They also participated in events outside Sydney such as the bus trip for committee members and their partners to establish a support group in the NSW country town of Orange. Among the travellers were some of Bill's early cochlear implant recipients, including the CICADA president at this time Alan Jones and a recent recipient named Neville Lockhart.

Neville was in his sixties and had grandchildren on the way when he decided to have a cochlear implant in 2005. He had relied on lip-reading for forty-five years and told Bill that he was surprised by how much he could now hear. As a young man living in Scotland, Neville had shied away from deaf groups, but not long after his switch-on, he decided to become involved with CICADA. This was after he had brought his wife Judy to their first Sunday barbecue and commented to her, 'They all seem so nice and normal'. Neville used his technical and organisational skills from a former senior scientist role with the CSIRO to contribute to the development of the CICADA website and the glossy magazine *Hearing HQ*.

CICADA had recently acquired its own club room at the SCIC. In addition to a cash donation towards the renovations from retailer Dick Smith, other donations included paint for the walls in a 'delightful' shade of lime green and trestle tables from Bunnings Hardware. John Boyle, a committee member who was born deaf and had used Sign Language before his cochlear implant, hand-carved a sign for the clubroom door and an elaborate wooden box which Bill thought looked 'a bit funereal', so he asked him, 'Have you made that to put my ashes inside?' John said, 'No, it's for the donations'.

Sue Walters and Bill had both noticed that more people from the Signing Deaf community were turning up to CICADA barbecues and making enquiries about having a cochlear implant at the SCIC. Bill had recently implanted a young Signing Deaf couple, Timothy and Angie Edwards, within a month of each other, because they wanted to be part of their eighteen-month-old daughter's hearing world. 'The day she was pointing to the trees at the laughing kookaburra was the day we decided to go for it,' said Timothy. 'We wanted to hear what Kiara was hearing.'[6]

After receiving criticism from the Signing Deaf community for so long, it was heartening for Bill to see attitudes to the cochlear implant changing. 'We received a battering from people who felt that Sign Language was their right and the cochlear implant was an invasion to their culture. No longer do they feel so threatened, which is wonderful.' In a complete turnaround, one Deaf group had even asked the SCIC for a donation for interpreter services.

Like the CICADA club room, the SCIC was also undergoing a facelift, but it was far more than a lick of paint. Chris Rehn played a crucial role in the renovation, which had a budget of $1.6 million and required the staff to move to the other side of the courtyard, above the new CICADA clubroom. As so often happens during a move, some precious items belonging to Bill were misplaced, including the silver cigarette case with little glass medicine vials inside which his father used on the battlefields during World War II. His father's microscope also disappeared, as did a large painting of three people on the beach at Dawlish which Bill had purchased during his last visit to see his father before he died.

When Bill was still living in London, he had treated the ears of several well-known racing car drivers, including Jackie Stewart, but there was not much he could do if they developed 'racing car deafness'. Bill was now able to offer a cochlear implant to one of the legends of the golden era of motorsport, eighty-year-old Sir Jack Brabham, who lived on Queensland's Gold Coast. Sir Jack believed that his hearing problems started in the 1950s, when his cotton-wool-and-wax earplugs offered little protection on the speedway and his ears would ring for days after a race. He came to Sydney for his cochlear implant operation after a chance meeting with Alan Jones in 2006, at the Phillip Island Classic Festival of Motorsport.

At this time there were three Sydney SCIC surgeons – Bill, Cathy Birman and Melville da Cruz – and three additional surgeons in Newcastle, where there was now a second branch of the SCIC: Kelvin Kong, Rob Eisenberg and Paul Walker. A clinical manager, Sharan Westcott, had been employed at the SCIC to prioritise the 300-plus implant surgeries undertaken by these six surgeons each year, of which Bill performed about half. The general manager of Cochlear Australia and New Zealand, Shaun Hand, commented: 'Prof was one of the top surgeons in the world at this time and the next highest group of surgeons were doing about sixty a year. Most surgeons do it as a sideline and average thirty per year, but Prof was doing five times that much. He would have done more if he could. He can't say no.'

When Bill reached his 1000th cochlear implant operation, a dinner was held at the Gladesville RSL Club, where he was presented with a spiral-bound album containing messages, photos and drawings from more than one-hundred adults and children. Some patients used poetry to express their gratitude, including nineteen-year-old Amelia Hardy, who had received her cochlear implant at two and described Bill as 'a brave surgeon, sent from above' (see poem, page 255). Chris Roberts presented Bill with a collector's edition bottle of Penfolds Grange Hermitage from 1984 – the year he started his program – to mark the significant achievement of implanting one third of *all* the people in Australia with cochlear implants.

* * *

If Chris Rhen was Bill's right-hand man during these busy growth years, then his left was Halit Sanli, who helps him with the electro-physiological testing and maintains a database of his patients. Since arriving in Australia, Bill has treated more than 1500 Menière's patients, which is one of the largest 'series' in the world. He has found there to be a 'bell curve' distribution of ages from nine to ninety, with a mean age for the onset of the disease of forty-eight. 'Menière's disease commonly strikes in mid-life,' says Bill, 'when people are typically at their most busy with family and careers.'

In addition to patients like Chrissy Boyce, whose Menière's symptoms built up over several years, there is a second group of patients who have no symptoms before their first attack. This was the case for 66-year-old Juliet Kirkpatrick, who was alone at home and in a distressed state when she rang her general practitioner to tell him the room was spinning violently. Bill was not surprised when Juliet told him that the manager of her security apartment block had to let her GP in because she was feeling so nauseous and vertiginous that she could not get up off the floor. Bill performed a controversial operation to remove, rather than drain, as some other surgeons do, the endolymphatic sac from Juliet's inner ear.[7] He believes that this procedure provides better relief from vertigo and reduces the tendency for recurrence several months or years after the surgery.

Bill is a world expert in Menière's disease and received the prestigious Clinical Gold Medal from the Prosper Menière Society in 1998. For many years Bill was both the patron and expert for the NSW Menière's Support Group, which was founded in the 1990s by Anne and Malcolm Stewart, with meetings in their home town of Bowral in the NSW Southern Highlands. At one meeting, Bruce Kirkpatrick discussed with Malcolm Stewart a paper he had read on Menière's and they pondered the question, 'What can we do about research into a cure for this disease, which is ruining the lives of our wives?' A doctor who was another founder of the support group, George Wilson, suggested they ask Bill to become involved and these discussions led to the formation of an entity known as the Menière's Research Foundation.

In 2001 Bill went with Bruce Kirkpatrick to see the dean of the Medical Faculty at the University of Sydney, Stephen Leeder, about setting up a fund within the university's Medical Foundation. Bruce is a successful businessman with good connections. Not only did he and Juliet personally pour thousands of dollars into this fund, but they encouraged others they knew to do the same. The Governor of New South Wales, Professor Marie Bashir, agreed to be the Patron-in-Chief of the foundation and was the guest of honour at a cocktail party held at Government House in Sydney on 23 September 2003 to thank their donors.

By 2007, the steering committee had reached the target of $300000 they needed to employ a suitably qualified and experienced research scientist. The process of finding the right person was no easy task, as inner-ear physiology is such a specialised field. Bill was impressed by a 28-year-old applicant from Perth, Daniel Brown, who was in the final stages of his PhD in the laboratory of a well-known physiologist, Robert Patuzzi.

Bill did not have the laboratory skills to train Daniel himself, but he knew an American research scientist named Professor Alec Salt, who is a world expert in the physiology of inner-ear fluids. Alec told Bill that he would be happy to have Daniel work in his Cochlear Fluids Research Laboratory at Washington University in St Louis, Missouri. During the next two years, under Salt's guidance, Daniel Brown learnt how to study ears with a disturbed flow and volume of endolymph – one of the fluids of the inner ear. Potassium-rich endolymph and sodium-rich perilymph are needed for the normal functioning of our inner ears, but in Menière's sufferers the inner ear and cochlea become engorged with endolymph in a condition called 'endolymphatic hydrops', which is thought to underlie the attacks of vertigo.

While Daniel was in the US, Bill was keen to continue his clinical research on patients with Menière's disease. This included a study which involved the injection of a contrast agent, gadolinium, through the tympanic membrane of the middle ear of patients and control subjects. Juliet Kirkpatrick agreed to be Bill's first volunteer and the day after the injection she underwent magnetic resonance imaging (MRI). However, the 1.5 Tesla MRI machine in the Radiology Department at RPA wasn't strong enough to replicate the subtle changes in the fluid volumes of the inner ear compartments Bill had witnessed during a trip to Japan.

During a week-long symposium held at the Nagoya University Hospital, Bill had been part of a group of of eight people who used contrast agent imaging to investigate the ears of three patients with Menière's Disease. The group was led by Professor Tsutomu Nakashima from the hospital's Department of Otolaryngology and Professor Shinji Naganawa from the Department of Radiology, which had a 3 Tesla MRI machine. By performing computerised analysis of a number of consecutive MRI scans it was possible for the group to make calculations of volumes and volume ratios of the endolymphatic fluid in the cochlea and vestibule.[8] This advanced MRI technology makes it possible to visualise the endolymphatic hydrops, a hallmark of Menière's disease, in a living person.

A Finnish otolaryngologist, Professor Ilmari Pyykkö, and Bill were the only non-Japanese members of the study group and their hosts wanted to show them something typically Japanese. After a train trip to the hot springs town of Gero, they went in a minibus up the side of the mountain to a traditional guesthouse, called a *ryokan*. Bill recalls that it was snowing and absolutely freezing the evening they ran outside and jumped naked into the hot tub in the men's bathing area of the guesthouse. During informal discussions on their return train journey to Nagoya, the group devised a simple three-stage diagnostic grading of the endolymphatic hydrops as 'none', 'mild' or 'significant'.

Bill believes in keeping grading systems for diseases as simple as possible. In the early 1990s, he developed a three-step clinical typing for the progression of Menière's disease, based on whether a patient's hearing was still fluctuating or they had become permanently deaf.[9] Around the same time he developed the 'Gibson Score', based on a set of ten questions clinicians can ask their patient, such as: 'Do you suffer from ringing in your ears? Do your ears feel full, like they would in an aeroplane?' If the person answers yes to seven or more of these questions, it is considered to be diagnostic of Menière's disease.[10]

The only female Graham Fraser fellow who came from the UK to be trained by Bill, Susan Douglas, mentions in her Fellowship report for the trustees that 'Prof' used the three-step staging and the Gibson Score during all his consultations with 'dizzy' patients.[11] During her six-month Fellowship, Susan and her husband announced they were expecting their first child and she was visibly pregnant in the photo taken of her with Bill and Alex in front of the sandstone walls at the entrance of the SCIC.

This was the same spot where a photo was taken of prime minister John Howard unveiling a silver plaque on 5 April 2007 for the official opening of the renovated SCIC. Bill says that John Howard was very open about his own hearing loss and enjoyed the tour of the new clinical facilities at the SCIC. Not long after the opening, one of the SCIC staff found a wooden box with an old brass microscope inside. Bill placed this microscope, which had once belonged to his father, on the deep windowsill of his freshly painted office.

During 2007, the SCIC employed Rob McLeod as their business manager. Rob was already well known to the staff as the father of Jack McLeod, who, as a toddler, had made quite an impression on *Midday with Kerri-Anne*. Now, a decade later, Jack's voice could be heard as part of the appeal for donations on the 2GB Radiothon, which raised $400000 for public patients to receive cochlear implants. Bill was one of several people interviewed on the day, between 5.30 am and 7 pm, by radio presenters Alan Jones and Ray Hadley.

Jack McLeod also featured on the cover of the *2007 Cochlear Annual Report*, running with two other boys along the edge of the surf, with a caption above his head: 'I'm just a normal kid with a bit of extra hardware'. Jack was old enough now to get to know his surgeon and describes Bill as 'a fantastic, inspirational person. Without him I might not have my hearing.'

* * *

The year 2007 marked twenty years since Bill had performed his first cochlear implant surgery on a child, Holly McDonell, whose photo has featured in several Cochlear brochures, including one giving a timeline of her personal achievements. Several Cochlear executives hosted an anniversary dinner for Holly near Circular Quay and they included on their guest list Bill and Alex, Chris Rehn and Holly's mother Viktorija, who had been inspired by her daughter's experiences to study for an additional degree and now works as a coordinator of rehabilitation for Cochlear in central Europe.

That same year, Holly visited the SCIC to share the good news that she had graduated from the University of Sydney with First-class Honours in commerce and law. 'It was a great achievement,' says Bill. 'When I implanted Holly, the NSW Department of Education said she should learn Sign Language, because she had no hearing after her meningitis. I had to fight to be able to operate on her and it was justifying seeing her fulfilling her dreams.'

Holly's visit inspired the speech Bill wrote for an SCIC fundraising event held later the same day, called the 'Blue Soiree'. The band's name was Blue Inc and the 300 attendees were requested to dress in blue. As a twist on the theme, Bill said to Chris Rehn, 'Why don't we go as the Blues Brothers?' Adam Spencer introduced the parents of a baby girl named Ava, whose two cochlear implants could now be managed by the clinical staff at the recently opened SCIC Canberra, saving them the stress of weekly visits to Sydney. Bill told the story of Holly McDonell's journey from being the world's first paediatric recipient of a bionic ear at age four to becoming a lawyer for Clayton Utz twenty years later.

Bill's UK fellow for 2007, Simon Freeman, attended the Blue Soiree and took his wife Mary, who was moved to tears by the personal accounts given on the night.[12] Freeman was the 12th fellow to be sent by the Graham Fraser Foundation, but the fund was by now depleted. The last fellow to be trained by Bill from the foundation was Neil Donnelly. He worked at Addenbrooke's Hospital in Cambridge with Bill's friend David Moffat, who says that he has trained just as many Australian fellows as Bill has trained British fellows. 'This reciprocal arrangement is largely because of our connection, so The London Triumvirate lives on.'

Like many of the other fellows, Neil Donnelly and his family rented a house on the Balmain peninsula so they would be near Bill and Alex, who became substitute grandparents to a league of small English children. Donnelly commented on how generous the Gibsons were as hosts, inviting his family to their home, beach house and to 'local eateries'. Bill also drove Neil around to their various clinical activities, including the Children's Hospital at Westmead, where they performed hearing tests on children every Tuesday and paediatric cochlear implants one Thursday per month.

Bill felt very privileged to be asked to perform a cochlear implant operation on the infant son of Pia Jeffrey. Pia's first child, Larissa, has normal hearing but her son Casey failed the SWISH test in the days after his birth. During more in-depth audiological testing, the clinic nurse confirmed the SWISH findings and then asked Pia, 'Do you have any family members who are deaf?' She replied, 'I am deaf', and then lifted up her hair to show the nurse her magnetised speech processor coil. Even the nurse in the maternity hospital had not been able to tell that Pia had a hearing impairment. Bill says, 'This is the little girl we were criticised for implanting at five years old. If anyone thought she would be able to speak like that as an adult, they would have said, "That's impossible."'

After one operating session at the Children's Hospital, Bill went out into the car park to discover that the hybrid engine of his Lexus had been alternating between its petrol and electric motor the whole time he was away. 'I must have got out and locked it with the smart key but not turned off the engine,' says Bill, who noticed afterwards that his fuel tank was nearly empty. Neil Donnelly relayed this story to Chris Rehn, who commented, 'Prof has just performed his first drive-through cochlear implant'. Neil says that Cathy Ball and Rose Ferris, who worked for Bill at his private consulting rooms in Newtown, would have him 'in tears of laughter' with all their 'Prof stories', including the one about the old lady who rang Rose to say she had left her glasses on Bill's desk. While Rose and Bill were rummaging through the papers on the surface of the Victorian writing desk, which had once belonged to his mother, Rose looked up to see a pair of bright pink spectacles perched on top of his closely cropped grey hair.

Every year in August Bill gave a talk to the medical students entitled, 'Hearing Loss in the Community'. To reach the Footbridge Theatre from his Newtown rooms, Bill walked along Carillon Avenue and through a set of entrance gates into the University of Sydney near the Women's College. He was not very far up the internal road when he developed chest pains with all the hallmarks of angina. He didn't want to disappoint the students, so he continued his walk to the theatre and gave the talk, but then rang a cardiologist named Ian Wilcox. An angiogram revealed two blocked heart arteries, so Professor Wilcox referred Bill to Strathfield Private Hospital, where an interventional radiologist inserted two stents.

By December 2008, Bill had recovered sufficiently from the stent insertion to fly to Germany to deliver the Sixth Memorial Wüllstein Address at the University of Wurzburg. After his presentation on Menière's disease, Bill met Wüllstein's much younger replacement as the head of the Department of Otolaryngology, Rudolf Hagen. During informal discussions with Hagen, Bill foolishly asked if Wurzburg had suffered much damage during World War II and Hagen replied, 'You British flattened it with your bombs!' Bill said in mock indignation, 'Hang on a minute. What about Liverpool and Coventry and Plymouth? They were all flattened as well.' This conversation brought back memories for Bill of the night he and John Tonkin had enjoyed a whisky with Horst Wüllstein at a men-only club in San Francisco eighteen years before.

* * *

Early in 2009, Daniel Brown returned from Washington and Bruce Kirkpatrick approached Professor Max Bennett at the recently opened Brain and Mind Research Institute in Camperdown about finding some laboratory space for this young researcher. Bill believes that the laboratory Bennett allocated to Brown is the only one in the world focused entirely on Menière's disease, rather than the physiology of the inner ear in general. There was a flurry of media interest about Brown's laboratory, including a radio interview with Dom Knight on ABC Classic FM.[13] In an article in *The Australian*, enitled 'Sound clues in mystery affliction', there is a photo of Brown in a white laboratory coat with a female patient.[14] The photo was taken in Bill's private consulting rooms in Newtown, only a ten-minute walk from Brown's laboratory, and the 'patient' lying on the examination couch is Celene McNeill, the audiologist who performed the hearing tests for Bill's patients in these same rooms.

Celene was studying for her PhD in audiology and Bill was very excited about her idea for a clinical study which measured the hearing of Menière's patients between and during attacks using specialised testing equipment in their own homes. The findings of this study were 'a revelation' and disproved the popular theory that attacks are caused by the rupture of a fine membrane and the sudden release of endolymphatic fluid. This rupture would have caused a drop in hearing, because the fluid suppresses the function of the sensory hair cells in the cochlea, but the paper Celene published in *Acta Oto-Laryngologica*, with Bill and his Chilean fellow Mauricio Cohen as her co-authors, demonstrated that the hearing of the subjects remained unchanged during their attacks.[15]

It wasn't only this study that supported Bill's view that a membrane rupture is not the cause of the fluctuating hearing and attacks of vertigo in Menière's disease; Daniel Brown's meticulous research in the years ahead also supported many of his views, in particular Bill's theories regarding the movement of endolymph fluid during attacks of vertigo. 'Mine were only theories,' says Bill, 'so it is lovely to have some laboratory experimentation to support them.'

Bill thinks that one of the reasons a 'cure' for Menière's has been so elusive is that it now appears to be a syndrome with two main presentations, rather than a disease. The first group of patients, who have pre-existing hearing loss like Chrissy Boyce, most likely develop Menière's disease because a fragment of otolith blocks their endolymphatic sac, preventing it from draining properly, whereas patients like Juliet Kirkpatrick, whose attack is the first sign of their disease, are thought to have an abnormal immune response to a viral attack. Bill thinks that a future herpes simplex vaccine may prove a useful 'solution', or perhaps even a 'cure', for patients with this second presentation of Menière's disease.

English translations are available of Menière's four papers, including the one he delivered on a cold day in January 1861, at the

Imperial Academy of Medicine in Paris, which described the symptoms of a disease that would later bear his name.[16] However, Bill wanted to read them in their original language. With little knowledge of French apart from what he had gleaned from listening to Michel Thomas language CDs in his car, Bill set himself the daunting task of reading a book about Menière and his life's work.[17] He had been given a signed copy of this book by one of the authors, François Legent, at a meeting in Paris to celebrate the 200th anniversary of Menière's death. The meeting included a visit to the Montparnasse cemetery, in the city's 14th arrondissement, where Bill was so excited to be standing next to the grave of this great man that he forgot the time difference and rang Alex, who said, 'William, it is 3 o'clock in the morning. I am going back to bed'.

In December 2009 Bill and Alex attended 'Voices of Angels', at the Angel Place recital room in Sydney's CBD, to hear their eldest grandson Jack singing with an Australian youth choir, the Gondwana Voices. Another cause for celebration during this same festive season was the recent arrival of Bill and Alex's only granddaughter, Saskia, a sister to Hugh and Cate's sons James and Milo.

However, by Christmas, Bill found himself flat on his back after a bulging disk in his cervical spine, revealed on an MRI scan to be C8, became acutely painful after he reached up to install a light fitting. One of Bill's visitors during January 2010 was Bob, who had recently sold his very successful Burgess Rawson real estate business and retired. The brothers are very proud of each other's achievements in two very different fields. They shared a laugh about the times Bill's patients had gone up to Bob in the city to tell him their symptoms.

Apart from a few visitors to cheer him up, the saving grace this summer holiday was a television mounted on the wall, where Bill and his 'fishing buddy' Mike Cook could watch the Ashes cricket test together. It was raining heavily the night Mike fell down the back steps of the wooden holiday house and the whole place shook, but Bill wasn't able to get out of bed. Mike was bruised but not injured and Bill had a brass plaque engraved with 'Cook's Landing 4 January 2010', which he screwed to the side of the step where Mike's bottom had landed. This plaque will always remind Bill of the summer he lost twelve days of fishing and three days of treating his patients. Both were a terrible loss.

CHAPTER 15

Winds of change

Even if he stops operating, he won't
be sitting around twiddling his thumbs.
He'll be travelling, teaching and using
his mind to explore new technology.
If you say the name 'Prof' to me, I will
only think of one person.

Chris Rehn, CEO of the Royal Institute
for Deaf and Blind Children

When Stephen Broomfield and his family flew in to Sydney in January 2010, he had a gnome to give Bill, which was a present from Professor Richard Ramsden in Manchester. Stephen was aware that his new and former bosses were 'old sparring partners' from their days working together at the London Hospital.

A few years before commencing his Fellowship in Australia, Stephen heard 'a strange on-air conversation' between the two senior professors during a LION live surgical broadcast, which was streamed live with interactive access to over thirty locations worldwide.[1] Richard was performing an operation at the Royal Manchester Infirmary to remove an acoustic neuroma and Bill asked him a question from a video conferencing room at the SCIC, where about twenty staff had gathered to watch the surgery. Richard exclaimed, 'Gibson, is that you? I thought you were dead.' When the Eurohub moderators asked Ramsden to explain what he was doing, he said, 'I'll talk slowly with no big words so Bill Gibson can understand'.

Bill felt very fortunate that a numb little finger on his right hand was the only side-effect of his recent spinal surgery (foraminectomy). His surgery day at the Mater Hospital, which was every second Friday, typically started around 7.30 am, when he backed his white Lexus out of the garage. Bill picked up Stephen from Balmain and during the thirty-minute drive to Crows Nest they discussed the three, or sometimes four, cochlear implant surgeries on their Friday list. The banter for the day started when Bill ribbed David Kinchington, or 'Kinch' as he calls him, about the length of time he was taking to put the first patient under a general anaesthetic. Other regulars in the operating theatre were the scrub nurse Sister Carol Macdonald and the bioengineer Halit Sanli, who performs the intra-operative testing.

Most surgical teams use a company-recommended procedure called neural response telemetry (NRT), to test the integrity of the electrodes in the cochlear implant. Stephen Broomfield says that Bill had come up with about ten alternative names for NRT, including 'No Response Today' and 'Nasty Rotten Test'. Bill comments that NRT has improved a lot but that it was awful to begin with, so he and Halit established their own testing procedure, which they performed in addition to NRT and facial nerve monitoring.

Bill used surgical thread to secure the green surgical drape in position behind the patient's ear with what he called 'Halit's stitches' – because they 'were designed to keep Halit's fingers away from the surgical incision'. Towards the end of the operation, Halit lifted this green drape and placed a magnetic coil on the skin over the site of the implant to test if each of the electrodes could send messages up the brainstem to the brain. This test is called electric auditory brainstem response, or EABR. If Halit was taking too long, Bill asked him, 'How do you say "Hurry up" in Turkish?', and Halit replied, 'There are no such words in Turkish.'

The first operation was declared a success, because Bill and Stephen had been able to preserve the patient's hearing in the low frequencies. The candidacy requirements for a cochlear implant had broadened in recent times to include not only profoundly deaf people but also those who are severely deaf and not able to hear over the complete speech range. Bill and Stephen were conducting a study to compare the Cochlear 422 with other models, including the Cochlear Hybrid, to see which was better at hearing preservation.[2] If successful, this enables the patient to hear a more natural blend of sounds through a specially selected hybrid speech processor, including their own low frequencies, which are amplified if necessary through a hearing aid component in the processor.

Between the first and second implant surgeries there was a break for scones with jam and cream, and then a second break for a hot or cold lunch in the staff dining room between the second and third operations. Each operation takes approximately two to two-and-a-half hours, so if there were no hold-ups Bill was home by 7 pm. The day following the surgery, which was always a Saturday for the Mater Hospital patients, Alex was usually on hand to cut the knots from the bandages around the patient's head so Bill could check the site of the wound prior to their discharge.

One Saturday morning per month, when Bill wasn't discharging patients from the Mater, he manned the barbecue stall for his local Rotary Club. The Saturday that the adult specialist audiologist Monica Bray saw Bill on the stall outside Woolworths supermarket in Darling Street, Balmain, she said to herself, 'How incredible is that? What other high-flying specialist would cook sausages on the weekend?' She adds that Bill does a lot behind the scenes that is not about the recognition.

Monica believed that much of the focus at this time was on cochlear implantation in children. 'Children were already well looked after,' she says, 'but few centres around the world were considering over sixty-five year olds for cochlear implants. Prof believes in the adult implant program and the SCIC is leading the way with their elderly experience.' By 2010, the SCIC had performed cochlear implants on more than 300 people over the age of seventy, including twenty-eight recipients over the age of eighty.[3]

Sylvia MacCormick, the nonagenarian who had spoken a few years before at the Arabian Nights fundraiser, was a member of Monica's 'oldest old cochlear implant club', which had fourteen members in their late eighties or over. Unfortunately, Sylvia was no longer able to deliver Meals on Wheels in her little red car to the older residents of Mosman, but Bill remembers that she was still quite sprightly and Alex regularly saw her at Australian Ballet Company productions at the Sydney Opera House.

Monica attended the 100th birthday celebrations of several SCIC clients, including Hellen Gengoult-Smith, who Bill operated on in 1999 when she was eighty-nine years old. Helen died a few months after celebrating her 100th birthday, so she enjoyed eleven years with her cochlear implant. Bill says many studies have shown that older recipients like Sylvia and Hellen feel less social isolation after receiving their implant and have a decreased risk of falls and dementia.[4] Despite these potential benefits, there are many deafened adults whose hearing aids no longer provide a benefit, but are unaware that a cochlear implant may be an option. Bill thinks that it is 'all a matter of awareness' on the part of the hearing-impaired person, their doctor and the staff in the hearing aids clinics.

* * *

For Norman Heldon's ninetieth birthday celebration, he trekked with twenty members of his family the 10 kilometres from the Federal Pass to Katoomba in the NSW Blue Mountains, including the final climb of about a thousand steps up the side of the escarpment. When Norman was assessed for a cochlear implant the same year, he was feeling nervous about being knocked back, but Bill told him that his 'superb physical fitness and mental state' made him a suitable candidate. Norman first noticed he was going deaf in 1944, during his time with the Royal Australian Air Force in England. 'I was serving on bomber command and my seat on the Lancaster bomber was right next to the engines. When I came back to Australia a year later, my hearing gradually became worse.'

Bob Ross is thirty years younger than Norman, but he also believes that his hearing loss resulted from the impact of loud noise during his army service. Bob joined the Royal Australian Artillery Corp in 1965 at nineteen years of age. He says he was wearing no protective hearing equipment when the loud 'ack–ack' sound of light anti-aircraft guns 'unfolded before my ears'.[5]

Bob encountered no difficulties when he had his first cochlear implant, but after Bill performed the surgery on his second ear in 2010, the discharge nurse forgot to issue the remainder of the packet of prophylactic antibiotics. Fortunately Bill and Alex were among the picnickers at Towradgi Beach for the launch of a new CICADA group in the Illawarra region, south of Sydney, where a park bench needed to become an emergency table. When Bill removed the cotton wool and examined Bob's recently implanted ear, he immediately sent a fellow picnicker with a prescription to find the nearest pharmacy. It took quite a few courses of oral antibiotics, and an explant operation, before Bob's weeping *Staphylococcus* infection cleared and Bill could replace his cochlear implant. It was a good reminder of the value of following the protocols his team had put in place in the early days of the adult cochlear implant program at RPA.

When Bill received a request to meet with Bruce Robinson, the dean of the Sydney University Medical School, in March 2010, he wondered what it could be about. On the way to Robinson's office, Bill crossed paths with a vascular surgeon he knew from RPA, John Harris, who warned him, 'Be prepared for a shock'. Bill took a seat outside the dean's office. His appointment followed that of James May, who, like Harris, is an Australian pioneer of treating aortic aneurysms by the insertion of fabric-covered stents.[6] Bill and these two other senior professors each met with a representative from Human Resources and Robinson, who had been supplied with what turned out to be an incomplete summary of their publication records from a university database and no information on the other significant contributions they were making to their departments. Robinson said to each of them in turn, 'We're under pressure to reduce staff numbers, so could you consider retiring or going part-time?'[7]

This was not the university's finest hour. The three senior academics interviewed by Robinson that afternoon, and about three others, were each leaders in their respective fields of medicine – including Bill, who considered himself to be both academically active and actively training the next generation of ENT surgeons. Within three days of his meeting with the dean, Bill developed chest pains. He had a waiting room full of patients in his private rooms at Newtown when he placed a call to his cardiologist, Ian Wilcox, to say, 'I think we need to bring forward my next appointment until tomorrow.' Wilcox said sternly, 'Bill, leave your patients and meet me at RPA in ten minutes'. During the week Bill spent resting at home after the insertion of his third stent – the maximum he could have before bypass surgery was recommended – Alex rang the dean's office and admonished them for the way Bill had been 'stressed out'.

Margaret Throsby was relieved and delighted when Bill was well enough to make a second appearance on her ABC Classic FM 'Mornings' program, only weeks after his stent insertion.[8] This time he was speaking to Margaret about Menière's disease, interspersed with some musical choices, including a piece sung by his grandson Jack. Towards the end of the hour-long interview, Bill even did some spruiking for a charity dinner that he and the Balmain Rotary Club were organising to raise funds for further research into this condition. The fundraising barometer of the Menière's Research Fund had by now passed the $1 million mark and a Japanese research fellow, Yasuhiro Chihara, had been employed to assist Daniel Brown with his Menière's research at the Brain and Mind Research Institute.

The fellows who came from overseas to be trained by Bill gained experience in a range of surgical procedures – including the controversial endolymphatic sac removal operation, which Bill advocates for some Menière's patients, and cochlear implantation. Several fellows commented on how much they enjoyed the long car trips with Bill to visit the more distant SCIC centres because it afforded them the opportunity to have in-depth conversations about their respective careers. Bill and his latest fellow from the UK, Andrew Cruise, drove the four hours each way to Canberra to observe the first operation on a child by Peter Chapman, who is one of the two local SCIC surgeons, along with Tim Makeham.

* * *

Since the official opening of the Lady Mary Fairfax Centre in Canberra in 2009, the SCIC had undergone another rapid growth phase. A new centre was about to open in Gosford and another further up the NSW coast in Lismore was already on the drawing board. It was up to the general manager, Chris Rehn, to meet with the politicians, stakeholders and benefactors, but he liked to involve Bill in important meetings, describing him as 'a genius on all fronts'. One of these benefactors was Jenny Parramore, who had heard Bill being interviewed on 2BL during the radio appeal in 2007. In 2010 she contributed $3 million through the Parramore Family Foundation to establish the SCIC in Lismore. Bill thought this centre should be named the Parramore Centre, but Jenny was adamant that it should be the Professor WPR 'Bill' Gibson Centre, and in the end she got her way.

Although Chris played a crucial role in the negotiations for the Lismore centre, he was no longer the general manager of the SCIC when it opened its doors in February 2011. In hindsight, Bill wishes he hadn't given Chris such a 'glowing reference' or he might never have accepted the offer to become the CEO of the Royal Institute for Deaf and Blind Children (RIDBC), following the retirement of John Berryman.

A couple of months before his departure, Chris reflected on the thirteen years he had worked with Bill: 'It has been a fantastic run with Prof, who will be the notional heart of the SCIC until he dies. Even if he stops operating, he won't be sitting around twiddling his thumbs. He will be travelling, teaching and using his mind to explore new technology. If you say the name "Prof" to me, I will only think of one person.'

Chris considers that he has a close relationship with Bill, but he also admires the closeness between Bill and Halit Sanli, who some of the SCIC staff still refer to as 'the A team'. An Inner Ear and Cochlear Implant Conference in Bodrum, Turkey, provided an opportunity for Halit and his wife Leyla to show Bill and Alex the home they had built near the town of Guvendik. From the flat roof of the Sanlis' four-storey dwelling, Bill could see some goats walking single file out of the pine forest at the back. As he turned to admire the majestic view of the Bay of Izmir and the Aegean Sea,

Bill mused over the winds of change blowing at the SCIC. There was Chris Rehn's imminent departure and also the news that Mark and Tanya Carnegie had separated and planned to sell their two cottages in Bronte.

A new home for the multi-disability children and their teachers would be found at the War Memorial Hospital, quite close to the two cottages in Bronte. Chris Rehn arranged for the day-to-day running costs of the Matilda Rose Centre to come under the auspices of the RIDBC. This was one of the first tangible steps towards his goal of less fragmented provision of disability services.

Chris was only twenty-seven when he first came to work for Bill at the 'rather creepy' former psychiatric wing at the Old Gladesville Hospital, and he was around forty when he left the SCIC in October 2010, with its five modern state centres. During that time the cochlear implant had gone from being an option for profoundly deaf people to being an 'expected standard of care' for people with severe to profound hearing loss. As a result of the introduction of the SWISH program, an eighteen-month-old child brought to the SCIC for a cochlear implant assessment was now considered 'a late diagnosis'. Bill had once been told that his concept of early implantation was too bold, but it was now accepted wisdom.

A relatively new indication for a cochlear implant is unilateral (single-sided) deafness. A Newcastle woman, Carolyn Holden, had been told many times that 'she just had to live with the tinnitus in her deafened ear'. Bill says that Carolyn's 'unbearable tinnitus', which had a score of 64 out of a possible 104 (over 17 is not good), overshadows any hearing she has in her good ear. Bill's initial application to the Central Sydney Ethics Committee to perform a cochlear implant operation on Carolyn was rejected. A 'ray of hope' opened up when Bill heard about a tinnitus trial in Holland, for which he would need to use the MED-EL brand of cochlear implant from Austria, like the European surgeons in the trial.

At forty-six years old, Carolyn became the first person with single-sided deafness in New South Wales to receive a cochlear implant and Bill gave a talk entitled 'Carolyn's Diary' at several conferences. The diary, which had been compiled by her audiologist, Monica Bray, documents the golden moment when, five minutes after her switch-on with the MED-EL device, Carolyn could understand 95 per cent of sentences through her deaf ear while white noise from an iPod blared into her good ear. When she is wearing her cochlear implant, Carolyn's tinnitus is no longer audible and she can enjoy conversations with her husband Robert, even when he is sitting next to her in the car.

The same month as he performed Carolyn's operation at RPA, Bill's Friday list at the Mater Hospital happened to fall on 1 April. He decided to play a 'little trick' on the scrub nurse he had known for many years. Bill asked for a MED-EL device for his first operation and Sister Carol Macdonald seemed rattled when she told him, 'I didn't think you used that brand, so I didn't order it in.' Later in the day, Carol rushed into the operating theatre and exclaimed, 'Someone has just smashed into a Lexus in the staff car park!' Bill and the anaesthetist both looked up in alarm and asked, 'What colour is it? White or black?' The penny then dropped for Bill who said, 'Carol, isn't it a bit late in the day for an April fool's joke?'

Since the mid-1980s, Cochlear has been the global cochlear implant market leader, and the company is particularly dominant in Australia. Its two major competitors, MED-EL and Advanced Bionics, gained approval to sell their devices in Australia in around 2004 and 2010 respectively. Although Bill remained loyal to the Cochlear device during his career, he welcomed these competitors because he believes that it keeps each company 'on their toes'.

Current models of the cochlear implant are extremely reliable but each of the manufacturers mentioned above has encountered reliability issues at some time. After Cochlear released the CI512 model, which had a slim, flat package, they found a higher than expected rate of product malfunction. In her role as a clinical support officer for the SCIC, Sue Walters remembers that Cochlear handled the issue very well and were quick to respond by initiating a worldwide voluntary recall of the CI512 in September 2011. Bill says that Cochlear flew replacement stock of their previous Freedom range of implantable devices to implant centres around the world, so that no surgeries needed to be cancelled.

* * *

In October 2011, Bill attended the Asia Pacific Symposium of Cochlear Implants in Daegu, Korea. For many years he had sat on the organising committee and in 2007 he was the president when the conference was held in Sydney. His decision to delegate his committee position during the Daegu conference was one of the steps in Bill's plan to retire from his Chair of Otolaryngology at the University of Sydney in ten months' time, when he turned sixty-eight.

Bill arrived home from the symposium on a Saturday, but was determined to attend the 'Celebrating Monica' farewell barbecue the next day, organised by the CICADA volunteer support group. Bill says that Monica Bray is a special person who always went 'above and beyond' in her job as an audiologist at the SCIC and that she was missed when she accepted a job at Cochlear. After twenty-two years in the job, Monica says that she did 'a lot of crying' as she packed up her room and said goodbyes to all her 'heroes'. These included 95-year-old Norman Heldon, who gave an impressive rendition of 'The Man from Snowy River' from memory for attendees of the final Tuesday evening SCIC seminar for 2011.

Due to the efforts of SCIC staff, including the IT manager Steve Pascoe, these professional seminars were now broadcast live to several centres around New South Wales and it was possible for the staff at these sites to ask the speakers at Gladesville questions. Broadband internet was also allowing the SCIC to take their services to some neighbouring Pacific countries which did not yet have their own cochlear implant programs.

Three boys from Samoa – Anzac, David and Francis Jr – had already travelled to Sydney at different times for their cochlear implant surgeries, which were provided for free by the SCIC surgeons.[9] After being switched on at Gladesville, it was possible for the boys' post-implant habilitation to continue in their home country due to a process called 'remote mapping'. Utilising a sophisticated video conferencing system at Gladesville, the SCIC staff are able to literally 'move the computer mouse' on the table of the clinic in Samoa. Steve Pascoe comments that the equipment at the far end – which consists of a laptop, webcam and a special pod for connecting the cochlear implant – is quite straightforward and has been used for clients in locations ranging from Port Macquarie to Nairobi.

The SCIC also provided assistance to the Northern Territory (NT) so they could establish their own cochlear implant program. Prior to this program, at least half a dozen patients had needed to travel to Sydney for their surgery. This included a ten-year-old boy, Rafael Villamer, who was born prematurely in the Philippines and had been deafened by the cocktail of drugs used to treat his low platelet count. After his switch-on at Gladesville, Raf was able to recognise his name and took great delight at listening to the sounds of animals on wildlife clips on his computer.

Since performing Raf's first cochlear implant operation in 2010, Bill has flown twice to the NT to provide support for the ENT surgeons at the Royal Darwin Hospital, Hemi Patel and Graeme Crossland, both originally from the UK. Among the patients on the second surgical list for Patel and Crossland, with Bill in a supporting role, was Raf because he was having a second implant in time for high school. In addition to providing visits by their surgical and audiological teams to Darwin, the SCIC has also donated four Cochlear devices, each valued at $25 000.

As the number of cochlear implant recipients in Darwin grew, it was clear that they needed their own branch of the CICADA support group. The president, Sue Walters, flew up to Darwin for the first picnic, which was held at the Palmerston Water Park in 2012. This event was organised by one of Bill's cochlear implant recipients, Chris Blackham-Davison, who drives around Darwin with 'ME DEAF' number plates on his Toyota SUV.

The SCIC would later establish a permanent centre in Darwin, but initially they sent outreach teams to assist implant recipients and forged links with other providers of hearing services, including Arafura Audiology and the RIDBC, which had recently established a service for the families of deaf and/or blind children in the Northern Territory.

When Chris Rehn first became the CEO of the RIDBC, he had floated the idea with Bill of 'joining up', because the two charities they represented provided similar services. In 2012, Chris approached Bill and the new CEO of the SCIC, Rob Mcleod, for a more formal discussion about a merger. Bill and Rob had some initial misgivings, because they were worried that the SCIC would become the junior partner of the much larger RIDBC. Another concern was that the RIDBC was a children's charity, whereas the SCIC provided cochlear implants to people of a wide range of ages. Bill comments that 'any merger had to be on the right terms'.

* * *

The SCIC was by now the largest provider of cochlear implants in Australia and Bill was one of nine surgeons who collectively performed more than 350 implant surgeries each year across thirteen hospitals. The SCIC newsletter, *Stay Tuned*, also reported that under Bill's direction his cochlear implant program had implanted just over 3000 people between 1984 and 2012.[10] One of Bill's Friday lists at the Mater Hospital in 2012 included Betty Lam, who was having her second ear implanted. When Bill and Alex visited Betty on the Saturday morning, they informed her that she was Prof's 2000th implant surgery. Bill was told at the time that he was the first surgeon worldwide to reach this milestone with the Cochlear brand of device.

This number of surgeries was a nice career highlight to have 'under his belt' and Bill was also keen to participate in a LION live surgery. As the venue, he chose the operating theatres of the brand new Macquarie University Hospital, which have the latest in audio-visual equipment. The global headquarters of Cochlear had recently moved to the Macquarie University campus, where several other hearing-related service providers would soon be located, in a building called the Australian Hearing Hub.

You have to admire Bill's stamina. After performing cochlear implant surgery at the Children's Hospital at Westmead in the morning, he operated on an adult at Macquarie University Hospital in the afternoon so that the hospital's IT officer could ensure the recording equipment was working perfectly. Meanwhile, staff from the SCIC and Cochlear started gathering in the hospital's ground floor boardroom for drinks and finger food, in readiness for the evening surgery. This would coincide with the morning in central Europe, where operations were also taking place in Antwerp and Warsaw.[11]

Disaster struck late in the afternoon when Bill, Cathy Birman and their surgical team were told that they had to move to a different operating theatre and the hospital's IT officer had already left to go home. Those assembled in the boardroom were streaming live to Europe and the rest of the world. Meanwhile, Bill was upstairs feeling frustrated that no one could see him successfully preserve a patient's hearing in the low frequencies during cochlear implant surgery.

Several of Bill's friends and former colleagues from the United Kingdom were likely to have been watching the LION broadcast, and he would be catching up with many of them on two overseas trips he made during the northern hemisphere summer of 2012. One of these visits was for a dinner to celebrate the 50th anniversary of starting his medical degree at the Middlesex Hospital. Bill's friend from the Middlesex Rugby Club, Bernie Ribeiro, had been raised to the peerage so he had access to the House of Lords. Bill and Alex sat at the same table as Lord Ribeiro for the alumni dinner on the Friday evening and on the Saturday there were some talks and recreations of musical numbers from the Manic Depressives Christmas concerts in the 1960s.

On the Saturday evening of the Middlesex reunion weekend, Stephen Broomfield organised a very well-attended fellows' reunion dinner. Among the guests of honour were Graham Fraser's widow Patricia and a trustee of the Graham Fraser Foundation, John Graham. The dinner was held in a restaurant called Brown's, near Lincoln's Inn Fields, which is one of the bastions of the legal establishment in the United Kingdom. A highlight of the evening was when 'Prof' was placed in the docks for 'misdemeanours against the fellows'. The reality of course was that Bill had shown the fellows such kindness that they will never forget what he and Alex did for them all.

The same English summer, Bill saw Richard Ramsden and David Moffat at the British Academic Otolaryngology Conference (BACO). David had been the 'Master' of the previous BACO, held in Liverpool in 2009, where Bill was awarded a gold medal, and Richard was the Master of the current meeting in Glasgow. Bill remembers Richard being 'in his element' at the Robbie Burns night he organised for the conference speakers, during which he 'stabbed the haggis' and quoted Burns poetry in a strong Scottish accent.

The three former colleagues and their wives also spent a pleasant weekend at the Ramsdens' landscaped estate in south Cheshire. Bill affectionately referred to Richard's castle-like home as Gnome Hall, because of all the gnomes he has given him over the years. To coincide with his move to Oxford, Richard planned to give his gnome collection away to the man who fished in his lake, so the three friends had fun taking photos of each other with a couple of these china figurines propped up on a bar stool. Richard and David, with whom Bill has shared such an easy and deep camaraderie since the 1970s, also watched him blow out the candles on a cake to celebrate his sixty-eight birthday.

When Bill retired as the Chair of Otolaryngology at the University of Sydney in August 2012, he also retired from his public hospital duties. Cathy Birman, Melville da Cruz and Jonathan Kong took over his public operating lists and Bill continued to operate on private patients at the Mater Hospital.

His replacement as the head of the ENT Department at RPA, Associate Professor Glen Croxson, agreed to take over the three-day temporal bone workshops for ENT surgeons, which Bill viewed as 'a poisoned chalice', because they were so much work to organise. Croxson also commissioned a portrait of Bill, which hangs on a wall opposite the reception of the ENT Clinic on level eight of RPA. The artist, Gillian Dunlop, who is also a rhinoplasty surgeon, has been praised for her portraits of Professor Dame Marie Bashir, Dame Quentin Bryce and Professor David de Kretser.

Bill's portrait serves as a reminder of all the registrars he has trained at RPA, including Cathy Birman, Melville da Cruz, Glen Croxson, Jonathan Kong and Phillip Chang. The last four of these ENT specialists also undertook Fellowships at Addenbrooke's

Hospital in Cambridge with David Moffat, so they received a double dose of London Triumvirate wisdom.

The locality surrounding the University of Sydney and RPA had been Bill's stamping ground for nearly three decades. All of the departments he visited were in walking distance of each other and his private rooms in the Chancellory, where he enjoyed a good relationship with the specialists in adjoining medical suites, including David Pohl and Jonathan Ell.

After sixteen years of conducting clinics in Newtown, with patients who had often travelled for hours to see him, Bill decided to close these private rooms and rent the space to another specialist. He was sad to say goodbye to his medical secretary Rose Ferris, technician Cathy Ball and audiologist Celene McNeill, and took the three of them out for lunch in Balmain. It was time to declare the end of an era and work towards the second, more emotionally wrenching stage of his retirement plan, when he turned seventy.

CHAPTER 16

Three score and ten

You have lived just the seventy years which are the greatest in the world's history and richest in benefit and advancement to its peoples... What great births you have witnessed!

Mark Twain[1]

W hen Bill Gibson retired from his Chair of Otolaryngology he became Emeritus Professor Gibson, but he still retained his title as director of the SCIC. He took car loads of patient notes and possessions from his private rooms in Newtown to the SCIC, including a cute sign to add to the collection of the medical secretary, Stephanie Walker, who he jokingly calls 'Stiff' because, he says, 'That's how she and other New Zealanders pronounce her name'. In addition to providing secretarial support for Bill, Stephanie is the medical secretary for five of the SCIC's ten surgeons, which at this time included Bill, Cathy Birman, Jonathan Kong, Alex Saxby and Simone Boardman, who flies up to Sydney from Tasmania to perform paediatric cochlear implant operations at the Children's Hospital at Westmead.

The SCIC surgeons have many 'friends', as they refer to the politicians, individuals and organisations who provide assistance and funding for their patients to receive cochlear implants at public hospitals, including Westmead and RPA. Bill says, 'We feel very fortunate that every NSW Health Minister since Peter Anderson has provided funding for public cochlear implant recipients. We don't mind which side of politics they're on – Liberal or Labor – as long as they help us.'

Bill was very impressed when the current NSW Minister for Health, Jillian Skinner, pledged an additional $1 million for public patients to receive cochlear implants. This equated to twenty-four more children and four more adults in the 2012–13 budget and brought the annual allocation of publicly funded cochlear implants in New South Wales up to 124. Bill has always worked hard to secure funding for children from uninsured families, so it was heartening when Skinner stated that her mission as Health Minister was 'to ensure that every child who needs a cochlear implant is able to receive one as early in his or her life as possible'.[2]

Jillian Skinner made these comments to coincide with the official opening in April 2013 of a new SCIC centre in Penrith, which caters for cochlear implant recipients in Greater Western Sydney and beyond. One implant recipient who was delighted by the opening of this new centre is Melinda Vernon, the elite runner and triathlete from Springwood in the Blue Mountains. Melinda was born profoundly deaf and received her cochlear implant at six, which she says helped her to enjoy a normal social life as a child. In 2009, at the age of twenty-three, tiny Melinda won the women's section of the City2Surf. She believes that being deaf has fuelled her competitive nature, 'driving her that step further to achieve what she has'.[3]

Melinda can be seen in photos from the Penrith centre opening with Bill and the Governor of New South Wales, Professor Marie Bashir, who believes that the cochlear implant is one of the greatest medical advances in her lifetime. Bill has come to know Professor Bashir quite well through her patronage of both the SCIC and the Menière's Research Foundation. He enclosed with her thank you note for opening this new centre a Hilaire Belloc poem he thought she would enjoy, entitled, 'Lord Lundy, who was too freely moved to tears and thereby ruined his political career', which includes the lines:

> Sir! you have disappointed us!
> We had intended you to be
> The next Prime Minister but three:
> The stocks were sold; the Press was squared:
> The Middle Class was quite prepared.
> But as it is! . . . My language fails!
> Go out and govern New South Wales!

Reading Hilaire Belloc poetry to his grandchildren is a Gibson family tradition that has been passed down through several generations, and another is the construction of the model to be placed in the middle of the table on Christmas Day with little presents inside. Bill and his grandsons were quite adventurous one year and made a schnauzer, with grey felt for the dog's body and white fluff for its ears. There had been three miniature schnauzers roaming around the top deck of the beach house that Christmas, including Laura's dog Lulu, but since then Lilly had died from pancreatic cancer and Wolfie had moved with his owners to Denmark.

Early in 2014 Bill was very concerned about Bob, who had been diagnosed the previous year with non-Hodgkin's lymphoma. Bob needed a stem cell transplant and Bill offered to be a donor, but the staff specialist haematologist at Royal North Shore Hospital advised against it. Bill still rang and visited as often as he was permitted during Bob's two-week hospital admission. Bob's daughter Jenny asked Bill for some childhood photos of her father for the wall poster she was making to brighten up his room, where visitors had to be gowned up to enter. Bill provided some photos of himself and Bob as blond-haired toddlers for the collage and she asked, 'Which one is Dad?' Bill replied, 'The goofy one'. Jenny smiled and said, 'You both look pretty goofy to me'. Thankfully during the months following his discharge from hospital, Bob's health improved.

When Bill decided to give up his regular fortnightly Friday operating list at the Mater Hospital after twenty years, the theatre staff gave him a farewell party. In many ways it was just a normal Friday list, with Bill performing three cochlear implant surgeries, but there was a certain buzz in the air. Bill's anaesthetist for the day, David 'Kinch' Kinchington, wore a leopard-print theatre cap and Bill wore a bright blue cap adorned with baby dinosaurs which had been a gift from one of his UK fellows. During the buffet lunch in the staff dining room, Carol Macdonald presented Bill with a book about the history of the Mater Hospital and forgave him for the jokes he had played on her over the years.

The only problem with giving up your regular operating slot is that it can become quite difficult thereafter to book a casual theatre list. In the months leading up to Bill's seventieth birthday, there was a scramble of patients who insisted on having 'Prof' as the surgeon for their cochlear implant operation. Bill performed one of his last operations on the first patient he had treated after arriving in Australia. Lilia Facchetti-Smith has made appointments to see Bill most years since her first appointment in his office at the Blackburn Building, late in 1983. Over the years Bill says that Lilia had become 'deafer and deafer', until she finally acquiesced to his suggestion that she have a cochlear implant.

Just as it is a difficult decision for a person to have elective surgery for a cochlear implant, it was difficult for Bill to agree to proceed with a merger between the SCIC and RIDBC until all of his concerns had been allayed. The CEO of the RIDBC, Chris Rehn, says that a 'feeling of goodwill' is a critical ingredient in merger negotiations between not-for-profit organisations. He reassured Bill and the CEO of the SCIC, Rob Mcleod, that adult cochlear implant recipients would always be part of their client mix.

Of course the merger involved a lot more than reassurance. Rob remembers there being eighteen months of negotiations between senior members of the SCIC staff, SCIC board members such as Denis Calvert and the RIDBC before an agreement was reached. The general consensus was that the merger would be for the greater benefit of both organisations and their clients. In the May 2014 issue of the SCIC newsletter *Stay Tuned*, Rob signalled that the two organisations had started to finalise discussions about a 'more formal' relationship.[4]

* * *

Bill turned seventy on 11 June 2014 and Alex had reached the same age thirteen days before. Bill considers that seventy – or three score and ten – is a fine age to attain, although he comments that it was once considered 'the end of the road' in biblical terms. Bill's great friend and mentor Barry Scrivener had ceased operating when he reached the age of seventy and Bill decided to do the same, before his hands 'started to get shaky'. Unlike 'Scrivy', who retired completely, Bill would still be treating his patients at the SCIC and assisting in the operating theatres with patients who request his presence. These stints in the theatres would ease his feeling of loss at no longer operating solo.

The itinerary for Bill and Alex's seventieth birthday trip included a touring holiday in France with their old friends John and Astrid

Gibson. Their stay in Arcachon brought back memories of the summer the two families spent walking through the scented pine forest to the beach, after Bill had completed his electrophysiology course at the Institut Georges Portmann. Bill and Alex visited Professor Michel Portman, who was nearing ninety years of age, and his daughter Annie at their family holiday house. From France, Bill and Alex took the thirty-five minute flight from Bergerac to Exeter.

Astrid and John were still away when Bill and Alex stayed in their home in Exeter and borrowed their car to make day trips to old haunts around the south-west of England. They caught up with Bill's Epsom College friend Robert Dyke and his brother John at a pub on the border of Cornwall and Devon. Another day they had a cream tea in Dawlish and walked around the grounds of Bill's childhood home, although Whickham Lodge itself had been replaced about a decade before by a small complex of exclusive townhouses.

From Dawlish, Bill and Alex drove the 16 miles upland to Totnes. An early memory for Bill, which he says is 'indelibly written' on his brain, is the sound of bombers flying over his grandmother's house from an American air base which remained operational for several years after World War II. Parking his friend's car near the driveway of Lakemead in Maudlin Road, Bill stood gazing up at the house, uncertain if he should ring the doorbell. The owner walked around the corner of the house pushing a wheelbarrow, and Bill was able to tell him that he had been born in one of their upstairs bedrooms. Nigel Kelland said, 'You must be one of the twins?' He then smiled warmly and said, 'My wife Julia will be dying to meet you. Would you and your wife like come in for tea and have a look around?'

The couples enjoyed each other's company on the tour of the Kellands' home and walled garden. The interior of the house and the attic were all very familiar to Bill, but smaller than he had remembered, leading him to comment: 'Everything seems much bigger when you are a child'. The cedar in the garden opposite the reception rooms of the house had been chopped down and was now a carved wooden seat, but one of the original grapevines continues to thrive in the glasshouse, with its year-round temperate climate.

From Exeter, Bill and Alex caught the train to Heathrow and arrived home in Sydney to the news that the merger with the RIDBC had been made effective as of 1 July 2014. On 24 August, Bill helped Sue Walters cut a cake at the Sunday CICADA barbecue to celebrate the 30th anniversary of her cochlear implant operation and she asked him with a smile, 'Prof, shall we make a second incision?' The next day, Bill handed over his directorship of the SCIC to his deputy director Cathy Birman, during Hearing Awareness Week. Jillian Skinner was present for this ceremony at the RIDBC in North Rocks, as were benefactors such as Jenny Parramore, who was in a wheelchair and looking frail the day the SCIC officially became 'an RIDBC service'.

Chris Rehn asked Bill if they could meet in a coffee shop in Lane Cove to discuss options for his new title. Bill told Chris that if he remained working after a similar handover of directorship in France, he would be referred to as *l'ancien directeur* or *le directeur fondateur*. They decided on the second of these titles, 'founding director', as a way to keep honouring Bill for his significant contribution to establishing the SCIC. What Bill learnt over thirty years, Cathy Birman would need to learn far more quickly in her new role as medical director of both the SCIC and RIDBC.

Unlike attempts by other groups to take over the cochlear implant program Bill had created, he was very accepting of the current change of ownership and leadership, stating simply, 'It is the way it needs to be'. A few months after handing the baton to Associate Professor Cathy Birman, Bill was back at North Rocks one Thursday morning to deliver a eulogy for Jenny Parramore's memorial service.

He was feeling emotional that day, because Jenny symbolised the many generous people who had shared his vision for the hearing impaired and provided the funds to realise his dream of providing SCIC services where people need them most, including recent centre openings in Darwin, Liverpool, Wollongong and North Rocks.

The SCIC also has a clinic at the Australian Hearing Hub, opposite the global headquarters of Cochlear in University Avenue, Macquarie University, with a couple of staff members, including Amy Rehn. One of the first conferences held at the Australian Hearing Hub was an International Music Symposium, chaired by Associate Professor Melville da Cruz, whose involvement over many years with the NSW Doctors Orchestra, Musicus Medicus, has included roles as the first violinist and the concertmaster. Music was for a long time considered 'the last frontier' for a cochlear implant recipient to conquer, but it is something that many people now strive to enjoy. In addition to *Play School*–style music groups for pre-school-aged recipients, there are music appreciation groups for adults in several SCIC locations.

A great honour for Bill was to be invited to cut the yellow satin ribbon across the doorway of the Gibson Room, in the Cochlear Clinical Skills Institute on level four of the Australian Hearing Hub. This 'room' is actually a $2 million temporal bone laboratory, with ten dissection stations, each equipped with a microscope and recording equipment. Bill says that on the day of the official opening, the first temporal bone course was already taking place, for some Middle Eastern doctors. Sue Walters, one of the speakers at the opening, spoke about the obstacles Bill had faced in establishing a cochlear implant program. She commented afterwards, 'When you're in a position like his, people try to undermine you, but Prof is staunch. Some people may have given up, but not him.'

On the morning of the opening Sue had been fitted with two of the latest speech processors from Cochlear, the Nucleus Series 6, which she was told would automatically adapt to her hearing environment. After delivering her 'honouring Prof' speech, Sue was walking down University Avenue when she stopped to say hello to one of the audiologists from Cochlear, Emma Ramsay. There was a cement mixer pouring concrete for a new path nearby, and this audiologist with normal hearing was having trouble hearing what Sue was saying. For Sue, the loud abrasive sounds seemed to fade into the background, while her own voice and that of Emma rose above it. The same thing happened the next morning in a coffee shop on busy Canterbury Road near Sue's home in southern Sydney. She could hear the voices of the friends from her yoga class, but the sound of the traffic rumbling past the door wasn't as obtrusive as usual. When Sue recounted these events to her 21-year-old daughter Ruby, she said, 'Mum, you must have bionic hearing'.

* * *

Since Bill commenced his medical degree fifty-plus years ago, he has witnessed many medical discoveries that aim to lengthen our lives well beyond three score and ten. He has also witnessed a revolution in his own medical specialty of otology and has met most of the key figures responsible for this great period of change – particularly with regards to what can be done to assist the hearing impaired.

When Margaret Throsby interviewed Bill on ABC Classic FM in May 2010, he told her that he had decided to specialise in otology because the field was opening up so rapidly. Bill said that it was really only about fifty years ago that not much could be done for most ear conditions. Then Horst Wüllstein learnt how to graft ear drums and John Shea Jr performed the first successful stapedectomy to replace the tiny stapes bone in the middle ear with a Teflon prosthesis. Bill told Margaret that 'the most fantastic thing of all' was discovering that we can implant prostheses to make people hear. During this radio interview Bill said that he had to be careful not to offend members of the Signing Deaf community, who view themselves as a distinct cultural group, but he believes that to be born profoundly deaf is the most devastating handicap someone can have, 'because if you can't have your hearing, you can't develop speech communication'.[5]

One of Bill's patients, NSW Labor MP for Cabramatta Nick Lalich, told him about the Hong-Kong-born, Australian businessman Henry Ngai, who is currently halfway towards his aim of donating $15 million worth of hearing aids to people in developing countries.[6] Ngai has made a fortune from his company ABC Tissues, which makes the Quilton brand of toilet paper, and has established several charities. These include ABC Tissues Hearing Express, which gave away 40000 hearing aids between 2011 and 2015.[7] Bill is one of the medical professionals who has helped to make this possible through several overseas trip he has made, including one to Fiji with Bronwyn Carabez and her charity the Carabez Alliance to assist in the fitting and distribution of approximately 1700 of Ngai's hearing aids to adults and children in Suva. The hearing aids Bill distributed were valued at approximately $1800 wholesale, or $4500 retail in an Australian audiology clinic.[8]

Alex accompanied Bill on a separate trip to a poor region of the Yang province in China, organised by Nick Lalich and Henry Ngai, whose goal was to distribute 5000 hearing aids in three days. Assisted by a team of medical students, Bill helped to test and fit 1500 people with hearing aids on both the first and second days. On the third day Bill recalls there was practically a riot and police had to be brought in to close the doors of the university auditorium because people in the queue were worried that supplies would run out. Bill and Alex came home with sore throats due to the terrible air pollution in this populous part of China, where they found it difficult to see beyond the first sporting field of a kung fu academy they visited, which was attended by 93000 boys.

It was nice to have a little more time these days to devote to these worthwhile causes, but for thirty years Bill had been kept extremely busy with his academic and clinical commitments at the University of Sydney, RPA and the SCIC. Several of his key achievements during this period were recognised recently when he was one of four people to receive a citation at the 2016 Conference on Cochlear Implants and Other Implantable Auditory Technologies. In front of an audience of 1500 conference delegates at the Sheraton Centre in Toronto, Canada, Bill received an Outstanding Achievement Award from the American Cochlear Implant Alliance and the University of Toronto, for: 'Lifelong leadership and staunch advocate for the implementation of cochlear implant technology in the treatment of the severely hearing impaired. Early proponent for universal neonatal screening using evoked response technology. Proponent for the establishment of easier access by virtue of multiple implant centres in Australia.'

One of the world's leading cochlear implant surgeons, Joachim Müller, had been the congress chair of this conference two years before, in June 2014. Professor Müller invited Bill to speak about the development of his 'small, straight incision' – which has been hailed as a major breakthrough in reducing the rate of surgical wound breakdown from as high as one in a hundred cochlear implant recipients[9] down to practically zero.[10] During the keynote presentations of the same conference, three cochlear implant pioneers were invited to speak: Graeme Clark (University of Melbourne), Ingeborg Hochmair (MED-EL, Innsbruck) and Blake Wilson (Duke University, US). In 2013 they had jointly received the most prestigious American science award, the Lasker-DeBakey Clinical Medical Research Award, for the development of the modern cochlear implant.

As the first device to replicate one of our senses, the cochlear implant has been awarded many scientific prizes and has also been 'in the frame' during the past decade for the Nobel prize. In a recent talk Bill gave in Japan about the changing indications for the cochlear implant he cited the well-known quote, 'Success has many authors; failure is an orphan'. Several individuals and groups have claimed to invent the cochlear implant, but Bill believes that the French scientist, André Djourno, should receive some of the accolades, 'because he really set the scene during the 1950s for everyone else who followed'. Bill says that several groups made contributions to this field during the 1960s and 1970s, including those led by William House in Los Angeles, Claude-Henri Chouard in Paris, Kurt Burian in Vienna and Graeme Clark in Melbourne.

'What Graeme Clark and his team did was come up with an idea for a multichannel device that was better than anyone else's at the time. Graeme then had the good fortune to have Paul Trainor from the Nucleus Group agree to take on the project and produce a commercially viable device which was years ahead of its competitors,' says Bill, who feels very fortunate to have been able to benefit from the work done by Clark's team in Melbourne and Paul Trainor's team at Nucleus in Sydney.

* * *

Bill and the bioengineer Halit Sanli are the only remaining members of the RPA adult cochlear implant program. Some believe that Bill would have 'hung up his boots' years ago if Halit had retired, and vice versa. In his workshop next to the CICADA club room at the SCIC, 65-year-old Halit handcrafts the single-use 'golf club' electrodes, dipping the rounded tip in pure gold, ready for Bill to use in his electrocochleography work. They make a dynamic team, testing the children's hearing at the Children's Hospital at Westmead and conducting research projects, including a new clinical study on Menière's patients.

Bill is ecstatic that Daniel Brown has been able to create an animal model of Menière's disease in the guinea pig and can visualise the compartments of their inner ears using 3D imaging. It was for this fluorescent imaging work that Brown received the 2016 Senior/ Principal Research Fellowship – equating to five years' salary and expenses – from the Garnett Passe and Rodney Williams Memorial Foundation. This means that Brown's research is no longer as reliant on fundraising, which Bill says was always intended to provide the 'seed money' for the project. Bill composed the message to go inside the charity Christmas cards produced by the Menière's Research Fund at the end of 2015. The card has a painting on the front of a harlequin face with black eye patches, which depicts a Menière's sufferer. Bill points at the painting as he says, 'It *is* a grim disease'.

During the two clinic days Bill spends at the SCIC each week, it is obvious that he is still much loved and needed by the SCIC clients and staff. Audiologists bring recent cochlear implant recipients into Bill's office so he can check the healing of their surgical incision. One day he was asked to provide advice on an elderly woman whose scalp was red and inflamed near the contact point with her magnetic processor coil. When Cathy Birman pops into his office for a collegial chat or to use his microscope for ear examinations, she still refers to him as 'Prof', as she always has. Cathy now has a fellow trailing behind her everywhere she goes, just as Bill did for twenty-five years.

Bill and Alex are still in touch with many of his former fellows, who also contact each other. It was a surreal experience for many of them to be 'plonked' with their families for six months in Sydney, which they describe as a beautiful city to call home. Those fortunate enough to be taken up on a flight with the Royal Flying Doctor Service by one of Bill's very early fellows, Neill Boustred, were in awe of the logistical challenges of delivering medicine to outback Australia, but mostly they saved their accolades for Bill. Professor

Henry Pau from Spire Leicester Hospital, who interviewed Bill on board his boat in 2005 as they cruised around Sydney Harbour, stated in the article he wrote for *ENT News*: 'Bill "Mad Wax" Gibson is a warm and friendly man. He is a true innovative academic, a great surgeon and a very patient teacher.'[11]

In addition to the overseas fellows they sometimes include in their travel plans, Bill and Alex have several 'second homes' with friends in Europe, including Halit and Leyla Sanli in Turkey, John and Sandy Graham near the French Riviera, John and Astrid Gibson in Devonshire and David and Jane Moffat in Cambridgeshire. Richard and Gill Ramsden have already welcomed the Gibsons to their new home in Oxfordshire, where Bill noticed that there was 'a complete absence of gnomes'.

One day at the SCIC, Bill tried to keep a straight face while declaring, 'Alex is leaving me!' It transpired that Alex had embarked on a sixteen-day trip with their daughter Laura to Barcelona, to attend a singing performance by their grandson Jack, who was on his gap year before commencing university. It was the longest that Bill and Alex had been apart since meeting at the age of twenty-one.

Other events involving grandchildren that feature on their social calendar include representative rugby games in country towns and 'playdates' with little Saskia, who is now in primary school. Since becoming a grandparent, Bill is aware of how much his own mother did for them all when he and Alex took their children down to Dawlish for family holidays. Bill thinks of his parents on special days during the year such as 18 October, which was not only John Gibson's birthday but is Physician's Day. It still makes Bill feel sad to think about his father's difficult death from oesophageal cancer and the tiny mouthfuls of Cornish pasty he was able to swallow during their last pub meal together at the Ship Inn. These painful memories, combined with the fact that his childhood home had been demolished, were for several years the reason Bill didn't want to return to Dawlish.

Despite having lived in Australia for over thirty years, Bill says that it is 'strange how your mind can flip back to where you came from when you are feeling stressed or upset'. On the way to a continuing medical education course at Concord Repatriation Hospital, Bill was in the process of changing a tyre in the pouring rain when he realised he had made 'the classic mistake' of forgetting to put on the handbrake. 'My beautiful Lexus rolled off the jack onto its nose,' says Bill, who asked the man who stopped to help if he could use his mobile to ring the AA – the UK Automobile Association. 'What's that?' said the man, thinking he wanted Alcoholics Anonymous. Similarly, when Bill's brother collapsed from heat exhaustion during a running event in Sydney's eastern suburbs in the 1980s, the race official asked for his address and Bob told him, 'Whickham Lodge, Dawlish'.

While Alex was in Barcelona, Bill dropped their latest miniature schnauzer, Willow, at the home of some friends in Balmain, and drove to St Ives to have a fiery curry and light beer with Bob at the Road to Goa restaurant. The brothers and their wives now see each other on a more regular basis and are planning to take a cruise together in 2018.

When Bill leaves the SCIC for the week, his once black briefcase bulges at the seams with the equipment he needs for his Thursday afternoon clinic at Celene McNeill's audiology practice in Bondi Junction. On such occasions, he is grateful for a lift to the car park at the bottom of Punt Road. During one of the final interviews for this book, Bill requested a lift instead to Balmain because his Lexus was 'in for a service'.

He provided directions to one of the Old Gladesville Hospital exits along an internal road which passes the sandstone graves of two former hospital superintendents, Eric Sinclair and Frederick

Manning. 'That's where I want my grave,' said Bill, pointing to the ornate, greying headstones. 'I've always fancied the idea of mourners holding umbrellas as they stand around a hole in the ground and throw dirt onto my coffin. Do you think Alex and Laura would come to place flowers on my grave every Saturday morning?' Bill then broke into one of his characteristic wide grins and it was obvious that he and Alex have made other plans.

Bill's story began in the middle of things, and it ends the same way. For the foreseeable future he will continue to combine his passions for travelling and teaching with treating the loyal patients who ring the SCIC to make appointments to see 'Prof'. The close connections he maintains and the joy that he brings to the lives of those around him are two of the qualities that endear Bill to his patients. This includes a young woman who describes these admirable qualities and his caring attitude in the closing poem. The ophthalmologist and humanitarian, Fred Hollows, once said: 'The basic attribute of mankind is to look after each other.'[12] The desire to help others still burns very brightly in William Peter Rea Gibson.

A tribute from a young patient

There was a brave surgeon, sent from above,
Who worked on my ears, and filled them with love.
With his nimble fingers, he took them from quiet,
Implanting a cochlear device, to make them hear right.

A long time ago, when I was five,
He found a good doctor, to keep me alive.
He stood by my bed, when diagnosed with a tumour,
And sent me balloons, with a great sense of humour.

This gift to us all is known as the Prof,
Who with endless devotion, kept the Ear Foundation aloft.
Thinking no one knows him, in fancy dress he takes great pride,
And at Christmas time, being a Santa he tries to hide.

I wish to say thank you, for helping me to hear.
It's with great gratitude, I hold you so dear.

Amelia Hardy

ENDNOTES

This section is for readers who wish to explore some topics in more detail. In addition to his book, *Essentials of Clinical Electric Response Audiometry*, Professor Gibson has authored or co-authored twenty-two chapters in books and more than one-hundred and thirty clinical papers. A selection of his important publications appears in these notes, as well as other sources of directly quoted material. Some of the notes include additional information which may be of interest to readers. The superscript numbers in the text are not intended to appear academic, but rather to facilitate the process of locating the relevant information in this section.

Preface

1. Graeme Clark. *Sounds from Silence*, Allen & Unwin, Sydney, 2000; Veronica Bondarew & Peter Seligman. *The Cochlear Story*, CSIRO Publishing, Victoria, 2012; and Mark Worthing, *Graeme Clark: the man who invented the bionic ear*, Allen & Unwin, Sydney, 2015.

CHAPTER 1

Memories of a father at war

1. Thomas Kelly. *The History of King Edward VI Grammar School Totnes and Its Famous Old Boys*. Totnes, 1947, p 60.
2. John Gibson. 'Family History by JH Gibson.' Gibson family private records.
3. The Charles Rea collection comprises fourteen lever arch folders in the Totnes Study Centre (at the rear of the Elizabethan House Museum) at 70 Fore Street, Totnes. The collection includes historical articles, sketches of the town layout and translations of documents (from Latin and Greek) going back at least three centuries. The collection was compiled and indexed in the 1920s and the town's historians are grateful because these documents survived the war while so many others didn't.
4. 'Death of Alderman CF Rea ... Three Times Mayor of Totnes ... A great loss to the Borough.' *Totnes Times and Devon News*, 16 March 1929, p 8.
5. John Gibson. 'The Phoney War.' Gibson family private records.
6. Christopher Murray. *Sean O'Casey: A Writer at Work*. Montreal, McGill-Queens University Press, 2004: p 280.
7. Paul Van Stemann. 'Himmler's night of reckoning.' *Independent on Sunday*, 21 May 1995: <www.fpp.co.uk/ Himmler/death/Wells_Independent_ Sunday.html>.

CHAPTER 2
Bill's school days

1. John Gibson. 'Family History by JH Gibson.' Gibson family private records.
2. Ibid.
3. Epsom College Education Trust and OE Club. *Carr House: Reflections of Members and Masters 1883 to 2011.* Self-published, 2011: p 8.
4. Index of Old Epsonian Biographies between 1915 and 1939. Doctors: GPs, Consultants and the Most Eminent.

John Hammond Gibson attended Epsom College from 1926–1930. He was a prefect, was selected for the Rugby XV and Cricket XI, and was awarded the MacFarlane Cup. He was the son of another old Epsonian, Dr William Gibson, who attended the College from 1895–1899: <archive.epsomcollege.org.uk/1915-1939/OE_Biographies/1915-1939.pdf>.

CHAPTER 3
A medical qualification

1. London Metropolitan Archives. Information Leaflet Number 34. Hospital Records, December 2010: <www.cityoflondon.gov.uk/things-to-do/london-metropolitan-archives/visitor-information/Documents/34-hospital-records.pdf>.
2. 'Lost hospitals of London: Middlesex Hospital, Mortimer Street, Soho': <ezitis.myzen.co.uk/middlesex.html>.
3. John Ezard. 'Queen Elizabeth, the Queen Mother.' *Guardian*, 31 March 2002: <www.theguardian.com/uk/2002/mar/30/queenmother.monarchy12>.
4. The workhouse in Cleveland Street was only nine houses from where Charles Dickens lived twice during his youth: <www.news.fitzrovia.org.uk/2013/06/10/plaque-unveiled-to-identify-charles-dickens-first-london-home/>.
5. University College London, 'Windeyer, history of a building 1959–2011', p 18. <www.ucl.ac.uk/sts/staff/reeves/outreach/Windeyer_project>.
6. Obituary: Sir Rodney Sweetnam. *Telegraph*, 9 July 2013.
7. CS Hallpike and H Cairns. Observations on the pathology of Menière's syndrome. *Proceedings of the Royal Society of Medicine* 1938; vol 31: pp 1317–31.
8. Memphis Public Library. 'Dr John Shea presents his professional papers to the Memphis Public Library.' Press release, 31 March 2013.
9. Jonathan Hazell. 'JGF: life and times.' Fourth Graham Fraser Memorial Lecture, 5 February 1998 at the Royal Society of Medicine, London: <www.grahamfraserfoundation.org.uk>.

CHAPTER 4
Fellow of the College of Surgeons

1. WPR Gibson. Avulsion of the upper limb. *British Medical Journal* 1970; vol 2: p 189.
2. 'Lost hospitals of London: Royal National Throat, Nose and Ear Hospital at 32–33 Golden Square': <ezitis.myzen.co.uk/rntnehgolden.html>.
3. Lord Macaulay wrote in 1685: '[it was] a field not to be passed without a shudder by any Londoner of that age. There, as in a place far from the haunts of men, had been dug, twenty years before, when the great plague was raging, a pit into which

the dead-carts had nightly shot corpses by scores. It was popularly believed that the earth was deeply tainted with infection, and could not be disturbed without imminent risk to human life.': <www.historic-uk.com/ HistoryMagazine/DestinationsUK/ LondonPlaguePits/>.

4. Royal College of Surgeons: Plarr's Lives of the Fellows Online. 'Hogg, James Cecil (1900–73)': <livesonline.rcseng. ac.uk/biogs/E005790b.htm>.

5. *Diseases of the Ear, Nose and Throat*, 2nd edition (in two volumes). Edited by WG Scott-Brown, J Ballantyne and J Groves. London, Butterworths, 1965.

6. Nick Black. A cradle of reform. *Journal of the Royal Society of Medicine* 2007; vol 100: p 177.

7. Lavinia Mitton. *The Victorian Hospital.* Oxford, Shire Publications, 2010: p 9.

8. WPR Gibson. The operating microscope and the development of ear surgery. *Journal of the Royal Society of Medicine* 1980; vol 73: pp 6–8.

9. R Dick, WPR Gibson and A Golton. A marker for middle ear tomography. *Journal of Laryngology and Otology*, 1973; vol 87, no 10: pp 1019–23.

10. WPR Gibson. A convenient method of examining the post-nasal space. *Journal of Laryngology and Otology*, 1972; vol 86, no 10: pp 1081–83.

CHAPTER 5
Taking a new direction

1. 'What is Menière's disease? Professor Bill Gibson explains.' Interview with Margaret Throsby on ABC Classic FM, 25 May 2010: <www.abc.net.au/classic/ content/2011/10/13/3337814.htm>.

2. G Portmann, GE Shambaugh Jr, IK Arenberg and CR Arenberg. The first inner ear surgery to conserve or improve a sensory hearing loss: A candid discussion of the first 50 years of endolymphatic surgery for hydrops with its innovator. *Revue de Laryngologie* 1978; vol 99, no 5–6: pp 277–98.

3. M Portmann, G Lebert and J-M Aran. Potentiels cochleares obtenus chez l'homme en dehors de toute intervention chirurgicale (Recording human cochlear potentials without surgical intervention). *Revue de Laryngologie* 1967; vol 88: pp 157–64.

4. Obituary: Madame Claudine Portmann. *Revista Brasileira de Otorrinolaringologia*, 2008; vol 74, no 2: <dx.doi.org/10.1590/ S0034-72992008000200002>.

5. RG Bickford, JL Jacobson and TR Cody. Nature of average evoked potentials to sound and other stimuli in man. *Annals of the New York Academy of Sciences* 1964; vol 112: pp 204–23.

6. E Douek, W Gibson and K Humphries. The crossed acoustic response. *Journal of Laryngology and Otology* 1973; vol 87, no 8: pp 711–26.

7. Jonathan Hazell. 'JGF: life and times', Fourth Graham Fraser Lecture, 5 February 1998, Royal Society of Medicine: <www. grahamfraserfoundation.org.uk/JGF life and times.pdf>.

8. 'Hallowell Davis, 1896–1992, a Biographical Memoir', by Robert Galambos, National Academy of Sciences, 1998: <www.nasonline.org/ publications/biographical-memoirs/ memoir-pdfs/davis-hallowell.pdf>.

9. Personal communication with Ellis Douek (email dated May 2016), and Douek's blog post 'Leave the deaf alone': <theficklegreybeast.squarespace.com/ journal/tag/ellis-douek>.

10. A Djourno and C Eyriès. Prosthèse auditive par excitation électrique à

distance du nerf sensoriel à l'aide d'un bobinage inclus à demeure (An auditory prosthesis through the remote electrical stimulation of the sensory nerve by means of an embedded device). *Presse Médicale* 1957; vol 65: p 1417.

11. Phillip Seitz. French origins of the cochlear implant. *Cochlear Implants International* 2002; vol 3, no 2: pp 77–86. Phillip Seitz was a historian for the American Academy of Otolaryngology – Head and Neck. To research the French origins of the cochlear implant Dr Seitz conducted interviews in America, followed by interviews in France in January 1994. The surgeon, Roger Maspétiol, was in poor health and declined to be interviewed, but it was possible for Seitz to interview André Djourno, Charles Eyriès and their laboratory assistant, Danièle Kayser. A version of this paper was presented at the Third International Congress on Cochlear Implants in Paris in April 1995. The investigations Seitz made in France were timely because Djourno and Eyriès both died in 1996.

12. WF House and J Urban. Long-term results of electrode implantation and electronic stimulation of the cochlea in man. *Annals of Otology* 1973; vol 82: pp 504–17.

13. 'Electronic ear aids the totally deaf'. *National Times*, 16–21 July 1973: p 37.

14. Graeme. Clark. *Sounds from Silence*. Sydney, Allen & Unwin, 2000: p 44.

15. John Graham. 'The French Connection: André Djourno and Charles Eyriès and the first cochlear implant. A tale of two pieds-noirs.' Presentation at the Auditory Prosthesis Conference, Asilomar Conference Centre, Monterey, California, 23 August 2003. Supplied by John Graham, Royal National Throat, Nose and Ear Hospital, Gray's Inn Road, London.

CHAPTER 6
The London Triumvirate

1. The Royal London Hospital Museum, St Phillip's Church crypt, in Newark Street, Whitechapel, London E1 2AD: <www.bartshealth.nhs.uk/rlhmuseum>. After the release of the David Lynch film *The Elephant Man* in 1980, starring John Hurt, the [Royal] London Hospital Museum scaled back the exhibit because of the hordes of tourists who flocked to see it. This included the removal of Joseph (sometimes referred to as John) Merrick's skeleton to the archives of the Hunterian Museum in the Royal College of Surgeons. During the same four years (1886–90) that Sir Frederick Treves provided care and accommodation to Merrick in a room at the rear of the hospital in Bedstead Square, Jack the Ripper murdered his victims. It was a commonly held belief among the ENT consultants during Bill Gibson's time at The London that this wealthy and eminent surgeon and Jack the Ripper were the same person.

2. TT King, WPR Gibson and AW Morrison. Tumours of the eighth cranial nerve. *British Journal of Hospital Medicine* 1976; vol 16: pp 259–72.

3. Nick Black. A cradle of reform. *Journal of the Royal Society of Medicine* 2007; vol 100: pp 175–79: <www.ncbi.nlm.nih.gov/pmc/articles/PMC1847731/>.

4. WPR Gibson. *Essentials of Clinical Response Audiometry*. New York, Churchill Livingstone, 1979: p 59.

5. WPR Gibson, DA Moffat and RT Ramsden. Clinical electrocochleography in the diagnosis and management of Menière's disorder. *International Journal of Audiology* 1977; vol 16, no 5: pp 389–401.

'In 65 per cent of the patients, a large DC potential was recorded which caused an apparent widening of the summating potential/action potential (SP/AP) waveform. This potential was thought to be an SP, which was enhanced relative to the AP component, and believed to be related directly to the presence of endolymphatic hydrops.'

6. WPR Gibson, RT Ramsden and DA Moffat. The immediate effects of naftidrofuryl on the human electrocochleogram in Menière's disorder (preliminary findings). *Journal of Laryngology and Otology* 1977; vol 91, no 8: pp 679–96.

7. WPR Gibson. Does electrocochleography still have a role to play in the diagnosis of Menière's disease? *ENT & Audiology News* 2012; vol 20, no 6: pp 67–69.

8. WPR Gibson and HA Beagley. Transtympanic electrocochleography in the investigation of retro-cochlear disorders.

Revue de Laryngologie 1976; vol 97: pp 507–16.

9. RT Ramsden, WPR Gibson and DA Moffat. Anaesthesia of the tympanic membrane using iontophoresis. *Journal of Laryngology and Otology* 1977; vol 91, no 9: pp 779–85.

10. JM Graham, RT Ramsden, DA Moffat and WPR Gibson. Sudden sensorineural hearing loss: electrocochleographic findings in 70 patients. *Journal of Laryngology and Otology* 1978; vol 92: pp 581–89.

11. RT Ramsden, DA Moffat and WPR Gibson. Transtympanic electrocochleography in patients with syphilis and hearing loss. *Annals of Otology, Rhinology and Laryngology* 1977; vol 86: pp 827–34.

12. DA Moffat, WPR Gibson, RT Ramsden, AW Morrison and JB Booth. Transtympanic electrocochleography during glycerol dehydration. *Acta Oto-Laryngologica* 1978; vol 85: pp 158–66.

CHAPTER 7
A major decision

1. GM Halmagyi, MA Gresty and WPR Gibson. Ocular tilt reaction with peripheral vestibular lesion. *Annals of Neurology* 1979; vol 6, no 1: pp 80–83.

2. WPR Gibson, PH Wade and W Oakes. Transtympanic electrocochleography or brainstem potentials – which is better for young children? Unpublished study conducted at the London Otological Centre, 66 New Cavendish Street, London W1.

3. DK Prasher and WPR Gibson. Brainstem auditory evoked potentials: a comparative study of monaural versus binaural stimulation in the detection of multiple sclerosis. *Electroencephalography and Clinical Neurophysiology* 1980; vol 50: pp 247–53.

4. RJ Black, WPR Gibson and JWR Capper. Fluctuating hearing loss in West

African and West Indian racial groups: yaws, syphilis or Menière's disease? *Journal of Laryngology and Otology* 1982; vol 96: pp 847–55.

5. British Society of Audiology. 'Recommended procedure for Hallpike Manoeuvre': <www.thebsa.org.uk/wp-content/uploads/2014/04/HM.pdf>.

6. Collegium Oto-Rhino-Laryngologicum Amicitiae Sacrum (CORLAS). 'Collegium history': <www.corlas.org/history/>.

7. Psychological and physiological acoustics: cochlear processes – in honour of Juergen Tonndorf. 120th meeting of the Acoustical Society of America. *Journal of Acoustical Society of America* 1990; vol 88, suppl 1: S122–23.

8. 'Cochlear implants (the bionic ear)':
    <stvincentsent.com.au/index.php/
    otology-neurotology-and-lateral-skull-
    base-surgery/cochlear-implant-the-
    bionic-ear/>.

9. David Pohl. 'Barry Scrivener AM,
    pioneer ear surgeon 1927–2000.' *Sydney
    Morning Herald*, 18 November 2000: p 91.

10. John Stubbs. 'The Silent World of
    J. Ashley, MP.' *National Times*, 9–14 July
    1973: p 37.

11. John Graham. 'The French Connection:
    André Djourno and Charles Eyriès and
    the first cochlear implant. A tale of two
    pieds-noirs.' Presentation at the Auditory
    Prosthesis Conference, Asilomar
    Conference Centre, Monterey, California,
    23 August 2003. Supplied by John
    Graham, Royal National Throat, Nose and
    Ear Hospital, Gray's Inn Road, London.

12. AC Coats and BR Alford. Menière's
    disease and the summating potential III:
    effect of glycerol administration. *Archives
    of Otolaryngology* 1981: vol 107, no 8:
    pp 469–73. The extra-tympanic ECochG
    method is also discusssed in WPR
    Gibson. *Essentials of Clinical Electric
    Response Audiometry*. New York, Churchill
    Livingstone, 1978: pp 90–93.

13. R Bannister, WPR Gibson, L Michaels
    and DR Oppenheimer. Laryngeal
    abductor paralysis in multiple system
    atrophy. A report on three necropsied
    cases, with observations on the laryngeal
    muscles and the nuclei ambigui. *Brain*
    1981; vol 104: pp 351–68.

14. Obituary: Sir Donald Harrison. *Telegraph*,
    15 July 2003: <www.telegraph.co.uk/
    news/obituaries/1436084/Sir-Donald-
    Harrison.html>.

CHAPTER 8

The new professor

1. 'Electronics will end deafness by year
    2000 – Professor', *Sounds News*, May
    1984, p 7. Reprinted from 'Predictions of
    Professor Bill Gibson', *University of
    Sydney News*, vol 15, no 32, 6 December
    1983.

2. Jane Hammond. 'Aboriginal children
    struck by silent epidemic.' *The Australian*,
    10 May 1990: p 5.

3. Professor Richard Dowell. 'Breaking
    the sound barrier: technology for the
    hearing impaired.' Presentation at the
    CICADA barbecue at SCIC, 5 June
    2011. Professor Dowell discussed the
    clinical trial at the Royal Victorian Eye
    and Ear Hospital in 1982 of the first six
    patients to receive the commercialised
    version of the Nucleus 22 device. He said
    there was such great variation among the
    outcomes of the first four patients to
    receive the device that he wondered if he
    needed to find a new career. However,
    the success of the fifth and sixth patients,
    combined with improvement in some of
    the first group of recipients, provided the
    impetus for Nucleus to launch larger
    trials in sites including: Sydney (Bill
    Gibson), Hannover (Ernst Lehnhardt),
    Houston (Herman Jenkins) and Iowa
    (Bruce Gantz).

4. Veronica Bondarew and Peter Seligman.
    The Cochlear Story. Melbourne, CSIRO
    Publishing, 2012: p 122.

5. Graeme Clark. *Sounds from Silence*.
    Sydney, Allen & Unwin, 2000: p 62.

6. Shirley Hanke. *The Story of CICADA*.
    Self-published, 2002: p 50.

7. Hanke. *The Story of CICADA*: p 53.

8. AQ Summerfield and DH Marshall.
    *Cochlear Implantation in the UK 1990–
    1994: Executive Summary and Synopsis*,
    MRC Institute of Hearing Research,
    University of Nottingham. Supplied by
    Dr John Graham, Royal National Throat,
    Nose and Ear Hospital, Gray's Inn Road,
    London.

9. 'The Bionic Ear ... a modern miracle.'
   New Idea, 12 January 1985: p 27.
10. Hanke. *The Story of CICADA*: p 29.
11. Hanke. *The Story of CICADA*: p 61.
12. 'Gail heard the bells', *Pacemaker: staff news sheet of the Royal Prince Alfred Hospital*, December 1985: p 3.
13. Royal Prince Alfred Hospital Audiovisual Department: video of cochlear implant operation on Susan Walters, 15 August 1984.
14. Clark. *Sounds from Silence*: p 161.
15. Hanke. *The Story of CICADA*: p 71.
16. Paulene Turner. 'A heart for a stranger.' 'Agenda' section, *Sydney Morning Herald*, 24 June 1986: p 17.

17. University of Sydney, Postgraduate Committee in Medicine, 'First annual postgraduate course on ENT disorders: a practical update for general practitioners', 23 November 1986.
18. The University of Sydney, Postgraduate Committee in Medicine. 'The surgery of the endolymphatic hydrops', 16–18 April 1986. Kaufman Arenberg demonstrated endolymphatic sac surgery, including the use of the Arenberg–Denver inner-ear valve/shunt (for endolymphatic hydrops), which was sold in the 1980s and 1990s by Hood Laboratories of Pembroke, Massachusetts, US.

CHAPTER 9
Children making headlines

1. John O'Neil, 'Holly's world full of sound again', cover story, *Sydney Morning Herald*, 9 July 1987.
2. Personal correspondence from the secretary of CICADA, Gladys Emerson, to the other committee members, 15 April 1986.
3. Jacqueline Leybaert. 'Effects of phonetically augmented lip speech on the development of phonological representations in deaf children.' In *Psychological Perspectives*, vol 2. Edited by Marc Marshark and M Diane Clark. Psychology Press (Taylor & Francis Group), New York, 1998: p 108.
4. WPR Gibson. 'Cochlear Implants.' In *Scott-Brown's Otolaryngology*, 5th edition. Edited by A Kerr and J Groves. London, Butterworths, 1987: p 615.
5. Kimberly Scott. 'Switched on for Life', *Daily Mirror*, 8 December 1989: p 3.
6. William Gibson. Graham Coupland oration: 'The ups and downs during the establishment of the Sydney Cochlear Implant Program'. Transcript of speech published in *Surgical News* January/February 2010: p 20.

7. Graeme Clark. *Sounds from Silence*. Sydney, Allen & Unwin, 2000: p 176.
8. Charles Pauka. The adult cochlear implant programme at the RPA audiology department in co-operation with the Department of Surgery, University of Sydney. *RPA Magazine*, Summer 1987: p 12.
9. Veronica Bondarew and Peter Seligman. *The Cochlear Story*. Melbourne, CSIRO Publishing, 2012; p 127.
10. Cochlear Australia and New Zealand website, timeline, '1987 First paediatric Nucleus Recipient': <www.cochlear.com/wps/wcm/connect/au/about/company-history>.
11. O'Neil. 'Holly's world full of sound again': p 1.
12. Graeme Clark. Speech made at Cochlear global headquarters, University Avenue, Macquarie University, 25 May 2012.
13. WPR Gibson. 'Cochlear implants in children: past, present and future.' Gordon Smyth Lecture. British Academic Conference in Otolaryngology (BACO), Liverpool, 8–10 July 2009.

14. 'History of deaf education.' Speech by Sharan Westcott at Australian Hearing in about 2005.

15. Clark. *Sounds from silence*: pp 180–81.

16. Jackie Allender. 'Voices raised against bionic ear.' *Weekend Australian*, 5–6 September 1987: pp 28–29.

17. Deborah Cameron and Yvette Steinhauer. 'First, waiting for a miracle. Then with the flick of a switch … Tears as Pia hears her first voice.' *Sydney Morning Herald*, 19 September 1987: p 1.

18. Personal communication with Prue Jeffrey (email dated 1 July 2016).

19. Chris Thomas. 'Hospital's savings earn bionic ears for 10.' *Sydney Morning Herald*, 31 July 1987: p 4.

20. Katrina Campbell. 'Alison ends her world of silence.' *Northern Star*, 6 November 1987: p 1.

21. Bondarew and Seligman. *The Cochlear Story*: p 127.

22. Michael Uniacke. 'Of miracles, praise – and anger – the Bionic Ear.' *In Future*, 1987; vol 6: pp 11–14.

CHAPTER 10
Storm clouds

1. Bruce Lee. 'Ear implant: a cure without a disease?', *Sydney Morning Herald,* 6 June 1990: p 2.

2. WPR Gibson and IK Arenberg, 'The Scope of intraoperative electrocochleography', in IK Arenberg (ed), *Proceedings of the Third International Inner Ear Symposium*, Kugler & Ghedin, Amsterdam, 1991: pp 295–304. This paper was presented at the Third International Symposium and Workshops on Surgery of the Inner Ear, conducted by the Prosper Ménière Society on 29 July – 4 August 1990 at Snowmass-Aspen, Colorado.

3. Leanne West. 'Now Andreas is back in touch with life again.' *Manly Daily*, 10 June 1988: p 1.

4. Veronica Bondarew and Peter Seligman. *The Cochlear Story*, Victoria, CSIRO Publishing, 2012; p 128.

5. 'Michael, David and Andreas are "$6m" kids.' *Glebe Weekly*, 9 November 1988.

6. Brett Wright. 'High-tech firm takes on the word.' *Future Age*, 1984, cited in Bondarew and Seligman. *The Cochlear Story*: p 230.

7. Obituary: Paul Trainor. 'Rare breed of native industrialist', in Jonathan King (ed), This Life, *Sydney Morning Herald*, 14-16 April 2006, p 24.

8. Bill Gibson. 'Farewell Paul Trainor'. *CICADA Newsletter*, July 2006: p 1.

9. Jane Southward. 'Bionics give gift of a toddler's cry.' *Sunday Herald*, 11 December 1988: p 25.

10. Personal communication with David Money (interview conducted in 2010).

11. Sydney University Children's Cochlear Implant Project. Submission to the NSW Department of Education, 12 May 1989: p 1.

12. Letter from Professor JA Young, Dean of the Faculty of Medicine, University of Sydney, to Professor WPR Gibson, 28 February 1990.

13. 'Electronics will end deafness by year 2000 – professor.' *Sounds News*, May 1984, p 9.

14. Kimberly Scott. 'Switched on for life.' *Daily Mirror*, 8 December 1989: p 3.

15. Letter from Government House, Canberra, to deputy vice-chancellor, The University of Sydney, Professor MG Taylor, 26 February 1990.

16. David McKnight. 'Fatal attraction: the academics who love steam.' *Sydney Morning Herald*, 8 August 1990: p 1.

17. Julia Patrick. 'Bill Gibson, cochlear implant hero.' *Quadrant*, June 2014, no 507: p 65.

18. Patrick. *Quadrant*, June 2014, no 507: p 65.

19. Catherine Brown, Maree Rennie and WPR Gibson. Case study: child with a surface electrode. Children's Cochlear Implant Centre (NSW), 1992.

20. 'Hearing breakthrough.' *North Shore Times*, 19–20 June 1992: p 1.

21. Deborah Smith. 'Deaf pride splits the silent world.' *Sydney Morning Herald*, 24 August 1991: p 7.

22. Norman Doidge. *The Brain that Changes Itself*, New York, Penguin, 2007: p 51.

23. WPR Gibson. Opposition from deaf groups to the cochlear implant. *Medical Journal of Australia* 1991; vol 155: pp 212–14.

24. Graeme Clark. *Sounds from Silence*. Sydney, Allen & Unwin, 2000: p 7.

CHAPTER 11

Casting the net long and wide

1. Memphis Public Library. 'Dr John Shea presents his professional papers to the Memphis Public Library.' Press release, 31 March 2013.

2. Victoria Campbell. 'Ear implants divide deaf community.' *Weekend Australian*, 22–23 August 1992: p 61.

3. Henry Pau. An interview with Professor William PR Gibson. *ENT News* 2005 (Nov/Dec); vol 14, no 5: <www.grahamfraserfoundation.org.uk/Henry%20Pau%20interview%20Gibson_ENT%20News.pdf>.

4. Personal communication with Roger Gray, Cambridge (email dated 28 June 2016). Dr Gray believes that the first child in the UK to receive a cochlear implant was a six-year-old boy, 'DB', who received a temporary electrode in an operation he performed at Addenbrooke's Hospital in Cambridge on 27 April 1986. It was DB's 'very positive' response to electrical stimulation which resulted in Gray's decision to operate on him a second time several months later as part of the UCH cochlear implant group, using their UCH/RNID cochlear device.

5. Sian Powell. 'Baby gets bionic ear implant.' *Sydney Morning Herald*, 17 December 1992: p 3.

6. S Aso and WPR Gibson. Electrocochleography in profoundly deaf children: comparison of promontory and round window techniques. *American Journal of Otology* 1994; vol 15, no 3: pp 376–79.

7. Graeme Clark. *Sounds from Silence*: Sydney, Allen & Unwin, 2000: p 162.

8. Obituary: Paul Trainor. 'Rare breed of native industrialist', in Jonathan King (ed), This Life, *Sydney Morning Herald*, 14–16 April 2006: p 24.

9. Louise Turk. 'Let's hear it for the Bionic Ear Man.' *Hornsby and Upper North Shore Advocate*, 14 June 1995: p 1.

10. 'Professor says thanks.' Letter to the editor from Professor William Gibson, *Hornsby and Upper North Shore Advocate*, 12 July 1995.

11. RL Webb, E Lehnhardt, GM Clark et al. Surgical complications with the cochlear multiple-channel intracochlear implant: experience at Hannover and Melbourne. *Annals of Otology, Rhinology and Laryngology* 1991; vol 100, no 2: pp 131–36.

12. WPR Gibson, HC Harrison and C Prowse. A new incision for placement of cochlear implants. *Journal of Laryngology and Otology* 1995; vol 109: pp 821–25.

13. Personal communication with Professor C Andrew van Hasselt, Faculty of Medicine, Department of Otorhinolaryngology, Head and Neck Surgery, Chinese University of Hong

Kong (email dated 21 June 2016). Bill performed two cochlear implant operations on 9 and 12 December 1994 at the Prince of Wales Hospital in Hong Kong. Andrew van Hasselt's team performed their first paediatric implant the year after this visit on 4 August 1995.

14. Fan-Gang Zeng. Cochlear implants in China. *Audiology* 1995; vol 34: pp 61–75.

15. Personal communication with Professor Jorge Schwartzman, Buenos Aires, Argentina (email dated 27 August 2015). In October 1993, Schwartzman invited Bill to deliver a presentation about

cochlear implants for the 150th anniversary of the British Medical Hospital. It was during this visit that they performed a cochlear implant surgery together.

16. 'Annita visits UKM's Medical Faculty'. *New Straits Times*, 17 January 1996: p 2.

17. Fax from Kevin Barry, Chief Barker of the Variety Club of Australia to Professor W Gibson, 26 June 1996.

18. Fax from Andrew Refshauge MO, Deputy Premier, Minister for Health, Minister for Aboriginal Affairs, to Professor WPR Gibson, 9 May 1996.

CHAPTER 12

A new centre and a new manager

1. Alex Gibson. Guest speaker at CICADA AGM 2007. *CICADA Newsletter*, March 2008: p 3.

2. Interview with Margaret Throsby on ABC Classic FM, 2 July 1998. Available to listen to on cassette in the State Library of NSW. Bill's musical choices: Beethoven's *Piano Sonata No 14*; Verdi's 'Chorus of the Hebrew Slaves' from *Nabucco*; Pachelbel's *Canon*; Chopin's *Funeral March*; and Tchaikovsky's *1812 Overture*.

3. *Midday with Kerri-Anne*, Channel 9, June 1997.

4. TE Mitchell, C Everingham, P Pegg, M Rennie and WPR Gibson. Performance after cochlear implantation: a comparison of children deafened by meningitis and congenitally deaf children. *Journal of Laryngology and Otology* 2000; vol 114: pp 33–37.

5. Peter Thompson. Interview with Jennie Brand-Miller on *Talking Heads*, ABC1 TV, 16 March 2009, transcript: <www.abc.net.au/tv/talkingheads/txt/s2511619.htm>.

6. 'The Ear Foundation 500th Cochlear Implant Celebration', *Weekly Times*, 17 May 2000: p 17.

7. Michael Goriany, '30 years of cochlear implants in Hannover', 20 August 2014: <www.lehnhardt-stiftung.org/2014/30-jahre-cochlear-implant-in-hannover/>.

8. Interview with Margaret Throsby on ABC Classic FM, 2 July 1998.

9. Shirley Hanke. *The Story of CICADA*. Self-published, 2002: p 1.

10. Colleen Psarros. Cochlear implantation in children who have additional considerations. *Sound Partnership* 2012; no 12: pp 6–7. *Sound Partnership* is an industry update produced by Cochlear Limited.

CHAPTER 13

The best use of the money

1. William Gibson and Richard Marshall. Obituary: John Hammond Gibson. *British Medical Journal* 2002; vol 324: p 429.

2. NSW Health. 'Guidelines: Statewide Infant Screening – Hearing (SWISH) Program', 12 February 2010. 'Significant

permanent bilateral hearing loss has an incidence of 1 to 2 per 1000 live births (approximately 80 babies in New South Wales per year). Significant hearing loss is defined as being greater than 40dB in the better ear', p 4. 'Infants who are admitted to Neonatal Intensive Care Units (NICU) are at a higher risk of moderate, severe or profound hearing impairment: 1 to 2 per 100 newborns': p 21: <www0.health.nsw.gov.au/policies/gl/2010/pdf/GL2010_002.pdf>.

3. David Leser. 'Bear in the boardroom.' *Sydney Morning Herald*, Good Weekend (supplement), 14 July 2012: p 24.

4. Peter Rea. Graham Fraser Foundation, Fellowship Report: <www.grahamfraserfoundation.org.uk/fellowship_report_rea.pdf>.

5. NSW Health. 'Background Paper: Universal Newborn Hearing Screening in NSW', June 2002. The chair of the Universal Newborn Hearing Screening Reference Group, Dr Elizabeth Murphy, held the role of clinical advisor, primary health and community branch at NSW Health. Among the sixteen members of the group were Professor Bill Gibson, Associate Professor Greg Leigh and Kirsty Gardner-Berry.

6. PA Rea and WPR Gibson. Evidence for surviving outer hair cell function in deaf ears. *Laryngoscope* 2003; vol 113: pp 2030–33.

7. NSW Health. *2004–2005 Annual Report of the Ministerial Standing Committee on Hearing (MSC-H)*.

8. Jaydip Ray. Graham Fraser Foundation, Fellowship Report: <www.grahamfraserfoundation.org.uk/Ray%20report.pdf>.

9. 'The Farrells are running again …'. SCIC newsletter, *Switched On*, June 2009: p 4. 'In what has become something of a tradition, Bradley and Thomas Farrell and a number of other SCIC supporters will be participating in the annual City2Surf in August.' Article includes photos of Team Farrell from 2003, 2004 and 2008.

10. Colleen Psarros. Cochlear implantation in children who have additional considerations. *Sound Partnership*, 2012; no 12: pp 6–7. *Sound Partnership* is an industry update produced by Cochlear Limited.

11. Shirley Hanke. *The Story of CICADA*. Self-published, 2002: p 73.

12. Constituency statement by Maxine McKew. House Debates, 2 June 2009: <www.openaustralia.org.au/debates/?id=2009-06-02.127.1>.

CHAPTER 14

Dreams becoming a reality

1. Menière's Research Fund, media release: 'Australian research could finally unravel the mystery of Meniere's disease', Sydney, 11 March 2009.

2. WPR Gibson. Menière's disease. *Otolaryngologic Clinics of North America* 2016/2017 (in press).

3. Chris Roberts. Transcript of speech made on 25 May 2005 at the launch of the Nucleus Freedom speech processor at the Museum of Contemporary Art, Sydney. *CICADA Newsletter*, July 2005: p 1.

4. SR Freeman, ME Bray, CS Amos and WPR Gibson. The association of codeine, macrocytosis and bilateral sudden or rapidly progressive profound sensorineural hearing loss. *Acta Oto-Laryngologica* 2009; vol 129, no 10: pp 1061–66. Paper presented by Monica Bray at the Audiological Society of Australia (ASA) State Conference in Perth in 2009.

5. 'Cochlear says let's hear it for local

legends.' *Inner West Courier*, 26 August 2008: p 34.

6. Denice Barnes, 'Parents make sound choice'. *Central Coast News*, 11 August 2004.

7. WPR Gibson. The effect of surgical removal of the extraosseous portion of the endolymphatic sac in patients suffering from Menière's disease. *Journal of Laryngology and Otology* 1996; vol 110, no 11: pp 1008–11.

8. T Nakashima, S Naganawa, I Pyykkö, W Gibson, M Sone, S Nakata and M Teranishi. Grading of endolymphatic hydrops using magnetic resonance imaging. *Acta Oto-Laryngologica* 2009; vol 129, supplement S60: pp 5–8.

9. WPR Gibson. The clinical typing of Menière's disease. In 'IK Arenberg (ed) *Proceedings of the Third International Inner Ear Symposium*'. Amsterdam, Kugler & Ghedini Publications, 1991: p 110. Presented at the Third International Symposium and Workshops on Surgery of the Inner Ear, Snowmass, Colorado, US, 29 July – 4 August 1990.

10. WPR Gibson. The 10 point score for the clinical diagnosis of Menière's disease. In 'IK Arenberg (ed) *Proceedings of the Third International Inner Ear Symposium*'. Amsterdam, Kugler & Ghedini Publications, 1991: p 109. Presented at the Third International Symposium and Workshops on Surgery of the Inner Ear, Snowmass, Colorado, US, 29 July – 4 August 1990.

11. Susan Douglas, Graham Fraser Foundation, Fellowship Report: <grahamfraserfoundation.org.uk/fellows/>.

12. Simon Freeman, Graham Fraser Foundation, Fellowship Report: <grahamfraserfoundation.org.uk/Simon%20Freeman%202007.pdf>.

13. ABC radio, *Conversations*, Dom Knight and Daniel Brown, 2 June 2009: <www.abc.net.au/local/stories/2009/06/02/2587343.htm>.

14. Helen Francombe. 'Sound clues in mystery affliction.' *The Australian*, 9–10 May 2009: <www.theaustralian.com.au/news/health-science/sound-clues-in-mystery-affliction/story-e6frg8y6-1225710599315>.

15. C McNeil, MA Cohen, WPR Gibson. Changes in audiometric thresholds before, during and after attacks of vertigo associated with Menière's syndrome. *Acta Oto-Laryngologica* 2009; vol 129, no 12: pp 1404–07.

16. Miles Atkinson. 'Menière's Original Papers: reprinted with an English translation together with commentaries and biographical sketch.' *Acta Oto-Laryngologica* 1961; Suppl. 162: pp 1–78. Based on the research by Miles Atkinson into how Prosper Menière spelt his own name, the author of this biography has decided to adopt the single grave accent over the second 'e' in his name. Prosper's son Emile added an acute accent to the first 'e' on his father's gravestone and to his name in the introduction to his journals, which were published in 1903.

17. F Legent, D Gourevitch, E Verry, AH Morgon and O Michel. *Prosper Menière: Auriste et Erudit 1799–1862* (Prosper Menière: Ear doctor and scholar 1799–1862). Paris, Flammarion Médecine-Sciences, 1999.

CHAPTER 15
Winds of change

1. Third Global Live International Otolaryngology Network (LION) surgical broadcast, 21 May 2008. The LION Foundation was created in 2006 as a non-profit organisation. The annual program offers participants

around the world direct and interactive access to international experts in the various fields of otolaryngology: <www.lion-web.org/pdf/2008_LION_flyer.pdf>.

2. W Gibson, H Sanli, C Birman and C Huins. Utilising intra-operative electrocochleography to assess the preservation of cochlear function during and after cochlear insertion. Presentation at the 14th International Conference on Cochlear Implants and Other Implantable Devices, Toronto, Canada, 11–14 May 2016.

3. Monica Bray. 'Practicing extreme audiology in an ageing society.' Presentation at the Australian Society of Audiology Regional Conference, Western Australia, 2009.

4. F Lin. Implications of hearing loss for older adults. *Audiology & Neurotology* 2012; vol 17, suppl 1: pp 4–6. Extended abstract from Aging and Implantable Hearing Solutions, Cochlear Science and Research Seminar, Paris, 19–20 March 2012.

5. Cochlear Awareness Network, 'Bob Ross': <www.cochlear.com/wps/wcm/connect/au/home/connect/personal-stories/bob-ross>.

6. Personal communication with Emeritus Professor John Harris (email dated 8 July 2016).

7. Personal communication with Professor Bruce Robinson (email dated 8 July 2016).

8. Interview with Margaret Throsby on ABC Classic FM, 25 May 2010. Bill's musical choices: Beethoven's *Moonlight Sonata*; Marta Keen's *Homeward Bound*, sung by Jack Begbie and his friend Jamie Carroll; *Deep Sea Dreaming*, by Elena Kats-Chernin, sung by Gondwana Voices; 'Jim' by Hilaire Belloc, set to music by Stephen Taberner and sung by The Spooky Men's Chorale; and Pachelbel's *Canon*. Podcast: <web.archive.org/web/20140125075652/http://menieresresearch.org.au/news/72-margaret-throsby-a-bill-gibson-on-abc-classic-radio-may-25th-2010>.

9. 'Taking SCIC services to the world', *Stay Tuned*, November 2010: pp 1–2: <www.scic.org.au/wp-content/uploads/2012/04/ST_10_Nov.pdf>.

10. 'A change of direction for Prof.' *Stay Tuned*, May 2012, pp 1 <www.scic.org.au/wp-content/uploads/2013/02/2012.-ST-May.pdf>.

11. LION 2014 – 9th Global Otology–Neuro-otology live surgery broadcast, 20 May 2014. Surgeries included in the broadcast: middle-ear surgery, middle-ear implantation, cochlear implantation, neuro-otology (i.e. removal of acoustic neuromas).

CHAPTER 16

Three score and ten

1. Mark Twain. Letter to the poet Walt Whitman, on the occasion of his 70th birthday on 24 May 1889. Reproduced in a letter from Alan Kohler of the *Australian Business Review* to Robert Gottliebsen on 30 December 2013: <www.theaustralian.com.au/business/business-spectator/letter-to-robert-gottliebsen/news-story/5eb44c4b3114c2f543e16f645f23e419>.

2. Jillian Skinner, NSW Minister for Health, media release: 'New cochlear implant centre for western Sydney', 23 April 2013.

3. 'Melinda watch: Melinda Vernon gold medallist and record holder.' *CICADA Newsletter*, Autumn 2010: p 7.

4. Rob McLeod, editorial: 'From the chief executive's desk', SCIC newsletter *Stay Tuned,* May 2014: p 3: <www.scic.org.

au/wp-content/uploads/2014/09/14.-
May-Stay-Tuned.pdf>.

5. Interview with Margaret Throsby on
ABC Classic FM, 25 May 2010. Link to
podcast of interview:
<menieresresearchaustralia.org/in-the-
media/>.

6. ABC Tissues Hearing Express website:
<www.abctissue.com/community.html>.

7. Hansard, Legislative assembly, 22 March
2016: pp 84–90.

8. 'Audiology training for locals', media
release, Fijian government, 16 August
2011: <www.fiji.gov.fj/Media-Center/
Press-Releases/Audiology-training-for-
locals.aspx>.

9. RL Webb, E Lehnhardt, GM Clark et al.
Surgical complications with the cochlear
multiple-channel intracochlear implant:
experience at Hannover and Melbourne.
Annals of Otology, Rhinology & Laryngology
1991; vol 100, no 2: pp 131–36.

10. William Gibson. 'The development of
the small incision for cochlear
implantation.' Presentation at the 13th
International Conference on Cochlear
Implants and Other Implantable Devices,
Munich, Germany, 18–21 June 2014.

11. Henry Pau. 'An interview with Professor
William Gibson.' *ENT News*, November/
December 2005; vol 14, no 5: <www.
grahamfraserfoundation.org.uk/
Henry%20Pau%20interview%20Gibson_
ENT%20News.pdf>.

12. Fred Hollows Foundation website, 'Fred
Hollows': <www.hollows.org/au/about-
fred#>.

SELECT BIBLIOGRAPHY

Samuel JMM Alberti. *Hunterian Museum at the Royal College of Surgeons Guidebook*. The Royal College of Surgeons of England, 2011.

Veronica Bondarew and Peter Seligman. *The Cochlear Story*. Melbourne, CSIRO Publishing, 2012.

Boyer Lectures. Robyn Williams in conversation with Professor Graeme Clark. Lecture 1: 'Exploring the world around us', 11 November 2007. Part of a series of six lectures entitled: Restoring the Senses. <www.abc.net.au/radionational/programs/boyerlectures/lecture-1-exploring-the-world-around-us/3210194>.

Graeme Clark. *Sounds from Silence: Graeme Clark and the Bionic Ear Story*. Sydney, Allen & Unwin, 2000.

Norman Doidge. *The Brain that Changes Itself: Stories of personal triumph from the frontiers of brain science*. New York, Penguin, 2007.

Epsom College Education Trust and OE Club. *Carr House: Reflections of Members and Masters 1883 to 2011*. Self-published, 2011.

June Epstein. *The Story of the Bionic Ear*. Melbourne, Hyland House Publishing, 1989.

WPR Gibson. *Essentials of Clinical Electric Response Audiometry*. New York, Churchill Livingstone (Medical Division of Longman Group Ltd), 1978.

WPR Gibson. 'Cochlear Implants'. A Kerr and J Groves (Eds) in *Scott-Brown's Otolaryngology*, 5th edition. London, Butterworths, 1987: pp 602–617.

Bill Gibson. 'Long Winding Road', CICADA BBQ 28 October, 2012.

William Gibson. Graham Coupland oration: 'The ups and downs during the establishment of the Sydney Cochlear Implant Program'. Transcript of speech published in *Surgical News* January/February 2010: pp 20–21.

WPR Gibson. 'Cochlear implants in children: past, present and future.' Gordon Smyth Lecture. British Academic Conference in Otolaryngology (BACO), Liverpool, 8–10 July 2009.

John M Graham. 'From Frogs' legs to Pieds-Noirs and beyond: some aspects of Cochlear implantation.' Graham Fraser Memorial Lecture, January 2002. <www.grahamfraserfoundation.org.uk/jgflect_2002_JMG.pdf>.

Shirley Hanke. *The Story of CICADA*. Self-published, 2002.

Julia Horne and Geoffrey Sherington. *Sydney: The Making of a University*. Melbourne, The Miegunyah Press, 2012.

Lavinia Mitton. *The Victorian Hospital*. Oxford, Shire Publications, 2010.
National Academy of Sciences. 'Sound from Silence: the development of cochlear implants' (Beyond Discovery series), August 1998. <www.nasonline.org/publications/beyond-discovery/sound-from-silence.pdf>.

Julia Patrick. 'Bill Gibson, cochlear implant hero'. *Quadrant*, June 2014, no 507: pp 64–65.

Margaret Throsby in Conversation with Professor Bill Gibson (about cochlear implants), ABC 702 Classic FM, 2 July, 1998. Available on cassette from the State Library of New South Wales.

Margaret Throsby in Conversation with Professor Bill Gibson (about Menière's disease), ABC 702 Classic FM, 25 May 2010. <www.abc.net.au/classic/content/2011/10/13/3337814.htm>.

Frederick Treves. *The Elephant Man*. London, Cassell & Co, 1923. Reprinted with commentary and illustrations in *Treves and the Elephant Man*, The Royal London Hospital Archives and Museum, 2003.

University College London. *Windeyer – history of a building 1959–2011*. <www.ucl.ac.uk/sts/staff/reeves/outreach/Windeyer_project>.

Whirled Foundation: Vestibular Disorders, A-Z Glossary of Terms. <www.whirledfoundation.org/wp-content/uploads/2015/10/A-Z-Glossary-of-Vestibular-Disorder-Terms.pdf>.

GLOSSARY OF TERMS

When our ears are working in perfect accord, our outer ears collect all the softness and loudness of life and set the process of hearing into motion. As long ago as the 6th century BC, the ancient Greek mathematician, Pythagoras hypothesised that sound was a vibration of the air and it was not long before people realised that these vibrations made the ear drum vibrate as well. Over the past one-hundred years, hearing aids have been introduced to alleviate mild-to-moderate hearing loss and in the past thirty or so years cochlear implants have been developed for people with severe-to-profound hearing loss. This glossary includes terms relating to hearing and balance, as well as their disorders and possible treatment with hearing aids and/or the cochlear implant.

Acoustic neuroma – is a tumour, usually benign and slow growing, which develops around the hearing and/or balance nerves. A mass forms due to the overproduction of Schwann cells, which make up the lining of the eighth cranial nerve. The neuroma can lead to gradual hearing loss, tinnitus and dizziness. These symptoms can be similar to those seen in patients with Menière's disease so a MRI or CT scan may be required to make a differential diagnosis.

Audiogram – is a graph for each ear which shows the levels of hearing. It can be described as a picture of your sense of hearing. There are several types of audiogram and audiometric testing including free field, speech, and pure tone, which is the most common.

Audiometry - pure tone measures the softest sound a person can hear across a range of frequencies in decibels (dB). The test involves the subject listening to a number of different pure tones through a pair of headphones and indicating if they can hear the tone. The top line of the graph (0 dB) represents perfect hearing. Today this zero level is determined with an artificial ear, set to an international standard, but in the past it was determined by testing an adequate number of people with no disorders of their ears or hearing. Hearing within normal limits is defined as someone who can hear very soft sounds between 0 and 20 dB HL (hearing level on an audiogram).

Auditory nerve – is also called the cochlear nerve and connects the inner ear to the brain. It forms part of the eighth cranial nerve which also contains the vestibular (balance) nerves.

Balance – is the sense we don't know we have until we lose it. The balance system allows someone to know where their body is in relation to the environment around them and maintain a desired position in that environment. The brain processes information from the vestibular apparatus (the organ of balance) and all the sensors in the body (including sight and touch) to maintain balance. If any part of this system is not functioning, then imbalance and dizziness may occur.

Bilateral – both sides, or both ears.

Bionic ear – is a popular name for a cochlear implant with multiple electrodes which provides hearing to people with severe to profound hearing loss. Professor Graeme Clark coined the term 'bionic ear' for the Australian-designed multichannel cochlear implant which has twenty-two electrodes, enabling sounds to be detected over the entire speech range.

Benign paroxysmal positional vertigo (BPPV) – is the most common form of dizziness and causes very brief symptoms, generally lasting less than a minute. It occurs when microscopic particles or crystals (such as fragments of the otolith organs in the inner ear) detach and find their way into the semi-circular canal. One form of treatment is a special manoeuvre to dislodge these particles. Sufferers experience the sensation of spinning, called vertigo, after making sudden head movements such as when they lie down at night, turn in bed and/or lift their head up. It is so named because it is not life-threatening (benign) and is also paroxysmal (occurs suddenly) and positional (occurs due to a change in position).

Cochlea – is a pea-sized structure, which is coiled like a snail's shell and embedded in the temporal bone. Approximately 3500 sensory (inner) **hair cells** line the two and three quarter turns of the fluid-filled structure. These hair cells translate a sound into nervous activity, which is sent via the auditory nerve to the brain. The adjective used to describe cochlea is cochlear.

Cochlear implant – is essentially an artificial inner ear, because it takes over the job of the damaged hair cells in the cochlea. It requires a surgical procedure to implant a hermetically sealed package of electronics called the **receiver–stimulator** under the skin, behind the ear. This package is connected to the **flexible electrode array**, which the surgeon inserts (usually through the **round window**) into the turns of the cochlea. The electrodes in this array convey bursts of electrical current pulses, which stimulate the adjacent nerve fibres. The first of the external components is the **speech processor**, which is sometimes called a sound processor. This battery-powered unit sits behind the ear like a hearing aid, and contains a **directional microphone** and electronics that process the sounds into digital signals. The speech processor is connected by a cable to the **transmitting coil** which transmits these digital signals

and power through the skin to the implanted receiver-stimulator and thus avoids the need for an implanted battery. The transmitting coil is held in place on the person's head by a magnet which aligns with a magnet in the receiver-stimulator.

Deafness – is the term used to describe a total loss of auditory function, whereas the term **hearing loss** should be used for people with a partial loss of function. However the terms are often used interchangeably.

Deafness/hearing loss - congenital is the term used to describe someone who is born with a hearing loss.

Deafness/hearing loss - acquired is the term used to describe someone who loses their hearing over the course of their lifetime, usually after the acquisition of speech and language.

Ear - outer is the ear canal and the external or projecting part of the ear, called the pinna (from the Latin for wing).

Ear - middle lies between the outer and inner ear. It contains three small bones of hearing (the ossicles) which conduct and amplify sounds for transmission to the inner ear or cochlea.

Ear - inner is the part of the ear that contains the organ of hearing (cochlea) and balance (the labyrinth and vestibule).

Electrocochleography (ECochG) – is a technique for recording the electrical potentials or signals from the inner ear in response to a sound. The results, which are recorded on an **electrocochleogram**, can provide evidence of Menière's disease and other ear disorders. The test involves the use of an electrode placed in the ear canal or alternatively a trans-tympanic needle or 'golf club' electrode placed in the middle ear.

Frequency – is the number of times sound energy oscillates in a second and is measured in Hertz (Hz). A sound with a low frequency will produce a low tone or pitch sensation, such as human heartbeat or bass guitar. Examples of sounds with a high frequency are a bird singing or a piccolo flute.

Habilitation – involves training sessions for cochlear implant recipients so they can learn to recognise the sounds generated by the speech processor in their cochlear implant. Congenitally deaf children and adults also need to learn how to understand speech, whereas those with acquired deafness may need to re-learn speech and language (rehabilitation). The duration of training is unique to the person and depends on their ability to adapt to the different sound sensations.

Hair cells – are the sensory receptors in the cochlea (and balance organs). They are topped with hair-like structures, called stereocilia, which move in response to waves of endolymphatic fluid in the cochlea. The mechanical energy of this movement is transformed by the hair cells into nerve impulses. When someone hears a high **frequency sound**, hairs cells near the **round window** entrance to the cochlea vibrate whereas low frequency sounds cause hair cells furthest away from the round window (apex) to vibrate. The hair cells are arranged tonotopically, i.e. like a piano keyboard. The same arrangement applies to the nerve fibres, which are stimulated by the hair cells, and also the auditory cortex of the brain where the message about the sound is finally received and processed into something meaningful.

Hearing – is the perception of sound in the brain. Hearing requires an intact cochlea, brainstem and auditory cortex. Only subjective hearing tests, which involve the cooperation of the person (such as pure-tone audiometry) can demonstrate that the entire system is functioning correctly.

Hearing loss - conductive is the inability of the middle ear to transmit sound energy, and therefore sounds, to the cochlea. This may be due to congenital abnormalities (i.e. a child born without an ear canal) or damage to the eardrum (i.e. due to chronic infections) or the tiny chain of three bones, called the **ossicles**, which can become either eroded or encrusted with bony tissue and therefore unable to vibrate. As a result, all sounds become fainter so hearing aids may be of use to people with this kind of hearing loss. Patients with **otosclerosis** have abnormal growth of bone in the middle ear and surgery can be performed to insert a prosthesis to replace the immobile stapes bone.

Hearing loss - sensorineural occurs due to pathology within the cochlea and less commonly from the nervous pathway leading from the cochlea to the brainstem. The main causes are ageing, Menière's disease, ototoxic damage, immune disorders and exposure to loud noise. People with sensorineural hearing loss find it more difficult to hear speech than those with conductive hearing loss. If their hearing loss is due to damaged sensory hairs cells within the cochlea but they still have sufficient auditory nerve fibres, they can be assessed as a candidate for a cochlear implant.

Hearing loss - mild is defined as someone who perceives their softest sounds between 20–45 dB HL. At this level, people can hear voices clearly in quiet situations, but they might have difficulty hearing soft speech at a distance or with background noise. Hearing aids are effective in treating mild hearing loss.

Hearing loss - moderate is defined as someone who perceives their softest sounds between 45–65 dB HL. At this level, people will find it difficult to follow conversations without some lip-reading, particularly if there is background noise. Hearing aids are effective in treating moderate hearing loss.

Hearing loss - severe is defined as someone who perceives their softest sounds between 65–90 dB HL. At this level, people cannot hear normal conversations and may experience difficulty even when using hearing aids, in which case they will be offered a cochlear implant.

Hearing loss - profound is defined as someone who cannot perceive sounds softer than 90 dB HL (and higher). It is sometimes called total hearing loss. Hearing aids are of no benefit and a cochlear implant may be an option.

Labyrinth – is a system of fluid-filled passages in the inner ear which consists of the cochlea, vestibule and semi-circular canals. The last two are concerned with our sense of balance and equilibrium. The bony portion of the labyrinth is made up of a series of canals formed within the temporal bone. Inside these canals is the membranous portion of the labyrinth. A fluid called the **perilymph** fills the space between the bony and membranous portions. The fluid inside the membranous portion is the **endolymph**. These two fluids play a role in the transmission of sound waves and the maintenance of balance. An excess of endolymphatic fluid can lead to a condition called **endolymphatic hydrops**.

Labyrinthectomy – involves the destruction of the membranous portion of the labyrinth to relieve frequent and debilitating attacks of vertigo, particularly in patients with Menière's disease. It destroys both the balance and the hearing so it is important that there is adequate balance function in the other ear. A non-surgical approach to selectively destroying the balance organ is the injection of ototoxic antibiotics such as gentamicin. Recently surgeons have combined surgical labyrinthectomy with a cochlear implant operation to restore the patient's hearing.

Mapping – is a term used for the programming of the speech processor for a particular cochlear implant recipient on the day of their switch-on. Mapping reviews are conducted at regular intervals for fine-tuning. The program, also called the **MAP**, is loaded into the speech processor by an audiologist, or other hearing professional, and instructs the software about how much electric current is required at a particular electrode to produce an audible, but comfortable level of sound. The MAP also instructs the external speech processor on how to select, reduce or enhance the sounds being captured by the directional microphones.

Menière's disease – was named for the Frenchman, Prosper Menière who in 1861 described a disease with the following cluster of symptoms: vertigo, tinnitus, varying types of hearing impairment and a feeling of fullness in the ear.

Nystagmus – is the term for rapid, involuntary, side-to-side movements of the eye, where movement to one side is slower than the other. It may be a sign of impairment of one of the semi-circular canals of the balance organ. Nystagmus is usually present during an attack of vertigo.

Ossicles – are found in the middle ear and are the three smallest bones in the human body. They play an important role in hearing by transmitting vibrations from the eardrum to the cochlea in the inner ear. They have distinctive shapes and are named after the Latin words for hammer (*malleus*), anvil (*incus*) and stirrup (*stapes*).

Otology – is the study of ears and an **otologist** is a medical specialist and/or surgeon who only treats disorders of the ear.

Oto-rhino-laryngology – is derived from the Greek for ear (*otos*), nose (*rhinos*) and throat (*larynges*), hence the term **otorhinolaryngologist** or **ENT** for a medical specialist or surgeon who treats ears, noses and throats. An **otolaryngologist** is a medical specialist and/or surgeon who only treats ears and throats.

Ototoxicity – refers to chemical-related damage of the sensory hair cells in the cochlea and balance organs. Ototoxic substances include quinine, codeine and certain antibiotics.

Round window – is the membrane-covered opening of the cochlea, which separates the middle and inner ear. The membrane is flexible, allowing wave-like movement of the endolymphatic fluid within the cochlea in response to vibrations of the stapes bone.

Speech perception - closed set is when a cochlear implant recipient repeats the test word or sentence from a restricted list of words or sentences (so there is a chance of guessing the correct answer).

Speech perception - open set is when a cochlear implant recipient repeats the test word or sentence without any visual or contextual clues (so there is no chance of guessing the correct answer).

Switch-on – takes places a week or two after the cochlear implant operation when the wound has healed and involves the activation of the device. The audiologist, or other hearing professional, first tests each of the electrodes in the cochlear implant to establish the threshold (softest level) and the maximum comfortable loudness level.

Temporal bones – are either of a pair of bones on the side of the skull, which enclose the ear canal, middle and inner ear. They are the hardest bones in the body.

Tinnitus – is a disorder in which sufferers experience the sensation of ringing, roaring and/or a buzzing sound in their ear(s) and/or head and is often associated with various forms of hearing impairment. Tinnitus is usually subjective; therefore can only be heard by the person with the disorder but cannot be measured precisely using any testing procedure. Objective tinnitus, which is rare, is due to sounds being emitted by the cochlea. Those who are eligible for a cochlear implant, due to their severe or profound hearing loss, often report that their tinnitus recedes or even disappears when their device is turned on.

Tympanic membrane – is the scientific name for the eardrum, between the outer and middle ear. It also isolates the middle ear from the ear canal, so no fluid can enter. It is part of the organ of hearing and vibrates in response to sound waves.

Unilateral – one-sided, or one ear.

Vestibular apparatus – is the organ responsible for our sense of balance. It consists of the utricle, saccule and three semi-circular canals, which lie within the inner ear. This apparatus provides information to a person about their posture, their movement and how gravity is affecting their body. Sensory hair cells in the fluid-filled, semi-circular canal move in response to movement and send signals to the brain that the person has moved in a particular plane (i.e. vertical, horizontal or diagonal).

Vertigo – is one of the main symptoms of a disordered vestibular system and gives the person the illusion of movement, such as the sensation of falling or the external world spinning. Brief attacks of vertigo are experienced by people with BPPV and prolonged attacks occur in sufferers of Menière's disease and vestibular migraine.

ACKNOWLEDGMENTS

I have always enjoyed true stories, or those inspired by true events, because they 'ring true' and are based on inspirational characters. Professor Bill Gibson is one such person and there were many people who considered him worthy of a biography, including the committee of the CICADA support group who commissioned me to write this book. A project of this scope necessitated the assistance of many people and I apologise in advance if I omit to mention anyone from the following pages.

From when I first met Bill and Alex Gibson in March 2009 it was obvious that they make a great team. Our lunch on their balcony, over-looking the marina, included fresh produce from the local Farmer's Market. When Alex expressed her disappointment at the free-range eggs on offer, I promised to bring eggs from my farm in the Southern Highlands to each of my future meetings with Bill.

It was wonderful to meet Bill's identical twin, Bob, at a coffee shop in the St Ives shopping centre. During an overseas trip I made to the United Kingdom in 2011, I was able to meet Bill's older sister Eleanor and her husband Richard, at their home near Northampton. Bob, Eleanor and Kathy have all been very generous in sharing their family story with me, as have all of Bill's family.

Jill Drysdale from the Study Centre in Totnes showed me the Charles Rea historical collection, and walked with me to Lakemead to introduce me to the current owners, Nigel and Julia Kelland, who invited me for morning tea. Likewise, Michael Yeo invited me inside Whickham Cottage in Dawlish which was the closest I came to imag-ining the presence of Bill's father, John and also his mother, Jane, who Bill mentioned several times was 'a similar size and shape' to me.

I am thankful to Bill's UK colleagues for helping me to build a pic-ture of his early career, including John Graham who I met at the Royal National Throat, Nose and Ear Hospital in London. John provided a personal introduction for me to visit the Royal College of Surgeons in

Lincoln's Inn Fields. The head of the conversation unit, Martyn Cooke, kindly showed me around the Hunterian Museum, their private archives and communicated with me by email about Charles Byrne's gigantism.

I doubt that many of the stories about The London Triumvirate, or even the chapter of the same name, would exist if I hadn't met with Richard Ramsden and David Moffat in Manchester and Cambridge respectively. I am indebted to Stephen and Clair Broomfield for having me to stay for two nights at their home Manchester and the stories Stephen told me.

These UK colleagues provided me with a perspective on Bill's international standing in ENT circles, as did two professors I met on my return journey to Australia. I had coffee with the Finnish otolaryngologist, Professor Ilmari Pyykkö in his beautiful apartment in Helsinki. In Nagoya I met with Professor Tsutomu Nakashima at the Nagoya University School of Medicine. Afterwards I had dinner with Professor Yoshiharu Masuda and Ryoko Asano, from Nagoya Gakuin University, who told me about a Skype-based cultural exchange between deaf teenagers in Japan and Australia. It was a rare privilege the following year to host three girls; Saya, Mizuki and Saeka, aged twelve, fourteen and sixteen respectively, on my family's farm. The girls also spent time in Sydney with several of Bill's cochlear implant recipients, including Sue Waters and Hisae Shibadai.

I am indebted to all of the SCIC staff for their assistance during my regular visits to the centre at Gladesville and especially: Sharan Westcott, Kirsty Gardner-Berry, Steve Pascoe, Halit Sanli and Stephanie Walker. I was fortunate to witness the inspirational work performed at the Matilda Rose Centre in Bronte by coordinator Maree Rennie, and her team of teachers. Maree also kindly continued our conversation over dinner at her home and contacted the Carnegie family on my behalf.

I am very grateful to Rob McLeod, the then CEO of the SCIC, for organising permission for me to visit two hospitals in late 2013. The first was the Royal Darwin Hospital where I met surgeons, Hemi Patel and Graeme Crossland, who took Bill, Halit and I out for dinner. Thank you also to Chris Blackham-Davison and the Villamer family for their hospitality in Darwin. It was a wonderful experience to be included in the farewell celebrations for Bill from the operating theatre staff at the Mater Hospital and speak to David Kinchington and Carol Macdonald.

Thank you to Professor Graeme Clark for our conversations and the tribute he wrote for Bill: 'The international success of the bionic ear is due to the scientists, clinicians and educationalists who worked in collaboration with Cochlear Limited. The sterling efforts of my colleague, Bill Gibson, over many years will make him a role model for other surgeons.'

Thank you to the following academics and learned professionals who responded to my questions and reviewed early drafts: Christopher Game, Michael Halmagyi, Henley Harrison, Cathy Birman, Melville da Cruz and Glen Croxson; Celene McNeill, Cathy Ball and Rose Ferris from the Newtown private rooms; Richard Dowell from the University of Melbourne; David Money and Peter Seligman about Nucleus; Theresa Spraggon, Judy Wimble and Sylvia Romanik about the children's cochlear implant program; Daniel Brown and Bruce Kirkpatrick about Menière's disease; John Harris, James May and Bruce Robinson from the University of Sydney; Philip Newall from Macquarie University; ABC 702 radio presenter, Margaret Throsby; businessman and Rotarian, Glenn Wran; current MPs, Nick Lalich and Jillian Skinner and the former MP, Peter Anderson who was very helpful. From the UK, thanks to Andrew Cruise, Neil Donnelly, Peter Rea, Henry Pau, Roger Gray and Ellis Douek, who provided translations for the French book and clinical paper titles. From the US, thanks to Irv Kaufman Arenberg, Alec Salt and Derald Brackmann.

The CICADA committee and members have also reviewed chapters. Thanks to Shirley Hanke for her useful collection of early photos and CICADA newsletters, and the current president, Sue Walters, for contacting other cochlear implant recipients on my behalf. To negotiate the path to publication of this book, Sue, Neville Lockhart and I formed a small editorial committee. This committee and CICADA are grateful to our two publishing partners for helping to make this book possible. At the Royal Institute for Deaf and Blind Children I wish to thank CEO, Chris Rehn for his great memory of dates and facts and also Professor Greg Leigh and Linda Berrigan for their assistance. At Cochlear Limited, I wish to thank Shaun Hand, Mark Salmon, Campion Fernando, Piers Shervington, Viktorija McDonell, Bern Ferraz and in particular Jim Patrick who read the entire manuscript and assisted with all my technical queries. Monica Bray has been very helpful with reviewing chapters and providing an audiologist's perspective.

Thank you to the following writers for reading drafts: Linda Emery, Sara Green, David Palmer and members of the Triune Writers Group. Despite all the assistance I have received, and my own best efforts, to err is human and any mistakes in the final manuscript are my responsibility. I welcome feedback to: www.tinaallen.com.au. During a manuscript assessment day at the NSW Writers' Centre, Helen Littleton from HarperCollins suggested several publishers, including NewSouth Publishing (NSP). I was delighted when the non-fiction publisher at NSP, Elspeth Menzies said in her acceptance email, 'With so much written on Graeme Clark, it's time for a biography of William Gibson!'

I learned so much from the dedicated team at NSP, who deservedly won Small Publisher of the Year in 2016. Thank you to Tricia Dearborn for asking the editorial questions that needed to be asked, and Susanne Geppert for her internal design and family tree. Luke Causby created the perfect clinical feeling for the book cover with his inspired blueprint of the inner ear. Thanks also to my project editor, Paul O'Beirne, who steered the whole publishing process with such consideration and expert care.

Elspeth Menzies has a flair for preparing a book for publication and suggested a foreword written by someone well known. Since my first conversation with Professor Dame Marie Bashir, I have found her to be a warm, special person, who has surprised and delighted me each time she has called to thank me or discuss something with me.

I would like to thank my family for being wonderfully patient and supportive, especially my husband David who has acted as a sounding board and read early drafts. My father Harold has always encouraged me in my studies and work. My children, James and Kaarina, are a constant source of joy and have spent a significant portion of their life living with this project so I thank them for that. My daughter was the one who said, 'Mum, just get on with it!'

Even though the writing of this book has been long, it has been richly rewarding. Soon Bill will be giving me my final Christmas card with 'thanks for the eggs' written inside. I will miss our meetings, which were more like fireside chats because Bill told me so many interesting stories about his family and the history of the British Isles. He introduced me to the poems of Hilaire Belloc, which I was thrilled to discover are now in the public domain. I have collaborated closely with Bill on every stage of this biography and I am very grateful to him for his frankness, willingness and good humour throughout the entire process.

Medical biographies don't generally include patient stories; however I knew they would be illuminating in many ways. I would like to thank the following people, and their families, for helping me to gain an understanding of what it is like to be hearing impaired and have a cochlear implant: Torben Albaek, Iskandar Alsagoff, Moisant 'Sonny' Bennett, Chris Blackham-Davison, Chrissy Boyce, the late Sir Jack Brabham, Professor Jennie Brand-Miller, Matilda Rose Carnegie, David Carter, Judy Cassell, Chris Connell, Anne Dernow, Zoe Dunn, 'Little' John Erdman Jr, Lilia Facchetti-Smith, Joseph Silipo, Jake Fisher, James Fletcher, Ruth Fotheringham, Joseph and Felicity Formosa, Amelia Hardy, Shirley Hanke, Norman Heldon, Carolyn Holden, Holly McDonell, Pia and Alex Jeffrey, Alan Jones, Lester Jones, Juliet Kirkpatrick, Neville Lockhart, Deborah Lee, John Lui, Ruby Loosemore, Hugh McCourt, Xanthe McLean, Holly McDonell, Jack McLeod, Cheryl Musumeci, Steve Pascoe, Bob Ross, Don Rouvray, Hisae Shibadai, Cathy Simon (later Easte), Teigan van Roosmalen, Alison Vary, Denise Venturini, Rafael Villamer, Melinda Vernon, Susan Walters, Roma Wood and Faye Yarroll.

Tina Allen

INDEX